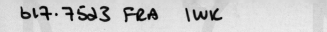

For Elsevier

Commissioning Editor: Robert Edwards
Development Editor: Kim Benson
Project Manager: Emma Riley
Design: George Ajayi
Illustrations Manager: Bruce Hogarth

Do5281

eye essentials

rigid gas-permeable lens fitting

Andrew Franklin BSc, FBCO, DOrth, DCLP
Professional Programme Tutor, Boots Opticians
Examiner, College of Optometrists, UK
Optometrist in private practice, Gloucestershire, UK

Ngaire Franklin BSc, FC Optom, DCLP
Examiner, College of Optometrists, UK
Optometrist in private practice, Herefordshire, UK

SERIES EDITORS
Sandip Doshi PhD, MC Optom
Optometrist in private practice, Hove, East Sussex, UK
Examiner, College of Optometrists, London, UK
Formerly Clinical Editor, Optician Journal

William Harvey MC Optom
Visiting Clinician and Director of Visual Impairment Clinic,
City University, London, UK
Professional Programme Tutor for Boots Opticians Ltd
Clinical Editor, Optician Journal, Reed Business Information, Sutton, UK

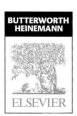

BUTTERWORTH HEINEMANN

ELSEVIER

EDINBURGH LONDON NEW YORK OXFORD
PHILADELPHIA ST LOUIS SYDNEY TORONTO 2007

ELSEVIER
BUTTERWORTH
HEINEMANN

© 2007, Elsevier Limited. All rights reserved.
First published 2007

ISBN-13: 978-0-7506-8890-1
ISBN-10: 0-7506-8890-4

British Library Cataloguing in Publication Data
A catalogue record for this book is available from the British Library.

Library of Congress Cataloging in Publication Data
A catalog record for this book is available from the Library of Congress.

Note
Knowledge and best practice in this field are constantly changing. As new research and experience broaden our knowledge, changes in practice, treatment and drug therapy may become necessary or appropriate. Readers are advised to check the most current information provided (i) on procedures featured or (ii) by the manufacturer of each product to be administered, to verify the recommended dose or formula, the method and duration of administration, and contraindications. It is the responsibility of the practitioner, relying on their own experience and knowledge of the patient, to make diagnoses, to determine dosages and the best treatment for each individual patient, and to take all appropriate safety precautions. To the fullest extent of the law, neither the publisher nor the editors assumes any liability for any injury and/or damage.

The Publisher

Working together to grow
libraries in developing countries

www.elsevier.com | www.bookaid.org | www.sabre.org

ELSEVIER   BOOK AID International   Sabre Foundation

ELSEVIER

your source for books,
journals and multimedia
in the health sciences

www.elsevierhealth.com

The
publisher's
policy is to use
paper manufactured
from sustainable forests

Printed in Europe

Contents

Foreword

Eye Essentials is a series of books intended to cover the core skills required by the eye care practitioner in general and/or specialized practice. It consists of books covering a wide range of topics ranging from routine eye examination to assessment and management of low vision; assessment and investigative techniques to digital imaging; case reports and law to contact lenses.

Authors known for their interest and expertise in their particular subject have contributed books to this series. The reader will know many of them as they have published widely within their respective fields. Each author has addressed key topics in their subject using a practical rather than theoretical approach, hence each book has a particular relevance to everyday practice.

Each book in the series follows a similar format and has been designed to allow the reader to ascertain information easily and quickly. Each chapter has been produced in a user-friendly format, thus providing the reader with a rapid-reference book that is easy to use in the consulting room or in the practitioner's free time.

Optometry and dispensing optics are continually developing professions, with the emphasis in each being redefined as we learn more from research and as technology stamps its mark. The *Eye Essentials* series is particularly relevant to the practitioner's requirements and as such will appeal to students, graduates sitting professional examinations and qualified practitioners alike. We hope you enjoy reading these books as much as we have enjoyed producing them.

Sandip Doshi
Bill Harvey

Introduction

It might seem a little eccentric to produce a book on rigid contact lenses when for the past 30 years their use has been in constant decline. When the authors entered contact lens practice in the mid-1970s, rigid lenses accounted for nearly all of the lenses fitted and soft lenses were the new kids on the block. At the time both the available soft lenses and their care systems were frankly not very good, but they have evolved to the point that most of the original advantages to RGP wear have been eclipsed. By 1991, RGPs accounted for 39% of lenses fitted in the UK and by the end of the 1990s leading figures in the contact lens world were predicting the virtual demise of rigid lens fitting by 2010. In 2001 only 7% of new fits were with rigid lenses, but they accounted for 21% of refits. However, the actual numbers of rigid lenses supplied does not seem to be declining, possibly due to the rise of planned replacement.

There are still considerable numbers of RGP wearers around, and anyone intending to practise as an optometrist should be aware of the basics of RGP fitting and aftercare. The UK General Optical Council (GOC) requires that those entering the profession should have both skills, and all training institutions for optometry retain RGP lenses on the syllabus. A number of factors have combined to make RGP lenses a difficult area for students and registered practitioners alike. The declining number of RGP patients is reflected in the experience available to undergraduate students in their clinics, and a significant number graduate with little or no practical experience of these lenses. The pre-registration year may offer little remedy, as some practices simply don't see many RGP patients. Many registered optometrists see few contact lens patients of any sort as, in large multiple practices, much of the contact lens work has been delegated to Dispensing Optician contact lens fitters.

This book is aimed at those entering the profession, as students, pre-registration optometrists or trainee contact lens opticians. Furthermore, those registered colleagues who are not in regular contact lens practice may find it of use as a refresher and update on current RGP practice, which has undergone an evolution of its own. It also aims to meet the requirements suggested in our new GOC entry level competencies to which all qualified practitioners are meant to adhere if maintaining their place on the GOC register. The authors have a combined experience of about 60 years of fitting RGP contact lenses (I suddenly feel old), and we have tried to concentrate on the practical aspects of selection, fitting and aftercare rather than obscure theory.

Dedication

To paraphrase the late, great Milligan: "After the last book, I swore I would never write another. This is it (or at least one of them)."

Acknowledgment

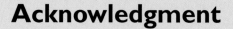

We are grateful to Chanel King and Heidi Harvey for assistance with photographs.

1
Initial consultation

Introduction

The initial consultation with a prospective contact lens wearer is an important dialogue between the practitioner and patient which has a number of goals:

1. To establish whether the patient is suitable for any type of contact lens correction.
2. To identify the optimal contact lens correction for the individual patient.
3. To establish reasonable expectations for the performance of the lenses and care system.
4. To educate the patient so that their use of the lenses will be safe and sensible.
5. To determine baseline information that can be used to monitor change that can influence future management decisions.

The majority of contact lens fitting is elective (i.e. non-therapeutic) and the patient will exert a degree of control over the lenses selected and their compliance with care systems. The principle of informed choice is important here. The patient must be given enough information to make appropriate decisions (i.e. those the practitioner approves of). The days when the practitioner held a monopoly on information have long departed. Most patients who present for contact lens fitting will also possess a computer and internet access. Therefore information that is incorrect or out of date will be easily detected, with consequent loss of credibility for the practitioner. It is important that practitioners keep themselves well informed on current developments.

Should this patient be wearing contact lenses?

There are few absolute contraindications to contact lens wear these days, though there are many more issues that may limit it or make it more complicated for the patient or practitioner.

Ophthalmologic consultation is essential before fitting any eye with active corneal pathology, and infective conditions should be eliminated before fitting to minimize the risk of microbial keratitis. The patient should be aware of any factors that will increase their risk so that they can weigh this against the benefits.

Ocular health

1. Ocular surface disorders may cause problems:
   (a) Recurrent erosions may be associated with anomalies of the basement membrane of the epithelium. In severe cases, a bandage lens may be indicated.
   (b) Recurrent bacterial infections will increase the risk of microbial keratitis significantly and in general these patients should be avoided.
2. Dry eye is the most commonly encountered complication. The effect on contact lens wear can be predicted by the severity of symptoms and corneal staining encountered before fitting. Patients with milder symptoms can usually be given contact lenses, at least for part-time wear.
3. Meibomian gland dysfunction (MGD) can be a significant factor in contact lens intolerance and its prevalence is age-related. Fewer than 20% of patients under 20 years of age present with it, but two-thirds of those over 65 years of age are found to have MGD.

General health

Both systemic pathology and the medication used to treat it may be significant factors when considering contact lenses.

1. Allergies may be associated with a poor tear film and a tendency to develop inflammatory reactions to solutions or lens deposits. Daily disposable lenses or non-preserved solutions may be indicated.
2. Patients with **chronic infections** such as sinusitis or catarrh may have excessive mucus in the tears. They may also be more prone to infection.

3. **Hypertensive** patients are prone to dry eye because of the β-blockers or diuretics used to treat their condition. A number of other medications have similar effects on the tear film. Common examples include antibiotics, antihistamines and psychomimetics such as diazepam, amitriptyline, chlordiazepoxide and thioridazine.

4. **Thyroid dysfunction** tends to cause both dry eye and poor blinking.

5. **Hormonal changes** associated with pregnancy, lactation and the menopause may be associated with a tendency to corneal edema and mucus accumulation. Generally it is unwise to commence fitting during pregnancy. The tear film may also be affected, and traditionally the use of oral contraceptives has also been assumed to have similar effects. However, a recent study (Tomlinson et al, 2001) did not support this assumption, possibly because modern contraceptive pills contain lower doses of hormone.

6. **Diabetic** patients may have a slightly higher oxygen requirement to avoid edema and an unstable refractive error. The cornea may be a little more fragile, and wound healing takes a little longer. However, a study by O'Donnell et al (2001) found that, provided the diabetes was well controlled, no extra risk was associated with daily wear. For extended wear, the reduced handling of lenses in insertion and removal might favor a fragile cornea, but there are insufficient data on complications with this modality, mainly because few practitioners are keen on anything beyond part-time wear. Daily disposable lenses are popular, but silicone hydrogels may give the best physiological response owing to their greater oxygen transmission.

Visual factors

A number of issues may be revealed by the patient's history:

1. Myopes will have a larger retinal image with contact lenses. This may improve Snellen acuity; however, it will reduce the field of vision a little.

2. Myopes who wear spectacles for reading may find they miss the base-in prism induced when they look through the near centers. The result can be a decompensated exophoria. Those who habitually read without spectacles will find that they have to accommodate more when wearing contact lenses. Those on the edges of presbyopia may struggle. Furthermore, the extra accommodation required will also cause extra convergence, which will tend to make the patient relatively esophoric.

3. Hyperopes will have a smaller retinal image with contact lenses. This improves their field of vision but may reduce their visual acuity. Many hyperopes only wear their spectacles for near vision tasks, and correction of their refractive error for distance may induce exophoria. However, hyperopic early presbyopes may find that contact lenses, particularly aspheric ones, help them read.

4. Prismatic correction is impractical in contact lenses unless it is vertical. For this, overall prism ballast can be used.

Psychological factors

The psychological traits of the patient may well influence their ability both to adapt to contact lenses and to look after them. A certain amount of intelligence is required to cope with lens care, preferably linked with a modicum of common sense. Extroverts may well adapt easily but can also become a little creative with their lens care since they tend to guess if unsure. Introverts may be detail-obsessed and find adaptation a challenge, particularly if they require exacting standards of vision.

Most elective fitting is driven by vanity, and the patient who is prepared to admit this will probably be honest about compliance after fitting. Some patients will invent spurious reasons for wanting lenses. The patient whose stated motivation involves the avoidance of fogging spectacle lenses may be just as evasive at their aftercare visits.

The perceived improvement in appearance that contact lenses may bring is a powerful motivation in many patients, particularly in those with high spectacle prescriptions. It may be even greater in those with iris anomalies, corneal scars or inoperable squints. It is often observed that such patients become more outgoing and optimistic when they wear contact lenses. However, there are some patients who expect contact lenses to improve an unhappy life, and they must be approached with caution. In all cases, the patient must have realistic expectations of what can be achieved. In general, a slight overstating of the difficulties likely to be encountered can be helpful. If the patient is anticipating some waiting around while you optimize the fit, they will not become anxious. If you sort things out more quickly than expected, the patient may think you are a genius.

It is worth bearing in mind that patients attending for sight tests have been found to have higher stress levels than those visiting the dentist. Contact lens patients have more reason than most to be nervous, so attention to phraseology and body language is important. Light-colored clothing may make the practitioner less threatening, and an informal manner also helps.

Occupation and lifestyle

There are some environments which are unsuitable or challenging for contact lenses, because of contamination or extremes of temperature. There are also certain occupations which discourage contact lens wear, sometimes on rather dubious grounds. Hygiene is always an important consideration, and a certain amount of lens handling is involved, during which rough or calloused hands may present a challenge to the lenses.

Financial considerations

There is a tendency to overemphasize this aspect, and practitioners sometimes offer lenses which are less than optimal on grounds of cost. Realistically, the average contact lens wearer probably spends more on a pair of shoes, and probably has more than one pair. Patients should be offered the best lens for their

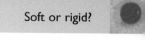

visual and physiological needs, and any compromise on financial grounds should be understood properly by the patient. Furthermore, a desire to save money on the lenses may also have implications for compliance with lens care.

Soft or rigid?

When the authors started fitting contact lenses this was a question that required some thought. Rigid lenses were more commonly fitted, as the soft lenses of the day were not particularly good. These days, however, soft lenses are the preferred option in most cases. There are lenses to fit nearly every patient and workable torics, multifocals and colored lenses are readily available. With the advent of silicone hydrogels, oxygen is rarely an issue and even extended wear is a practical proposition. Daily disposables even circumvent the chore of cleaning and storing the lenses. The biggest advantage of soft lenses, however, is that they are comfortable from the outset, unlike rigid lenses which require adaptation before acceptable levels of comfort are attained. In this world of instant gratification people are often not prepared to invest the time and effort to adapt to RGPs, but there are still some patients for whom RGP lenses should be first choice:

1. Patients with irregular astigmatism due to corneal damage or keratoconus will only attain satisfactory vision with RGP lenses.
2. Existing rigid lens wearers may not be satisfied with the visual performance of soft lenses.
3. Patients with particularly exacting visual requirements will probably see better with RGPs. This is particularly true for presbyopes.
4. High minus prescriptions will result in lenses that are thickest at the edge of the optic zone. On a hydrogel lens, oxygen transmission is likely to be poor. It will be better on a silicone hydrogel, but an RGP lens will give a much better oxygen level around the limbal area.

5. Patients who have limbal neovascularization from previous soft lens wear will be better off in RGPs, though silicone hydrogels are also an option.

Patient examination

The examination of the patient can begin as naked-eye observation during the initial dialogue. In particular at this stage look for the following:

1. Make a note of the patient's **complexion**. Patients with auburn hair and freckles tend to have more sensitive corneas.
2. Note **eye color**. Blue-eyed patients tend to be more sensitive, especially with rigid lenses.
3. **Lid position** will be important particularly with RGPs, torics and multifocals. If the lid position is unusual, a diagram should be drawn illustrating it.

The rest of the examination is conducted with the major slit-lamp. The examination has three phases:

1. General observation of the eye and adnexa.
2. General observation of the cornea with white light and medium magnification.
3. Specific examination of the cornea with white and cobalt blue light.

General observation of the eye and adnexa

General observation of the eye and adnexa with a low-magnification setting may be conducted with focal illumination and a wide beam, but often a far better view can be obtained by the use of diffuse illumination. The diffuser gives the effect of a much larger light source and gives the eye a more natural appearance, as well as allowing more of the eye to be illuminated at one time. Shadows tend to be minimized, allowing detail to be seen. On the other hand, some loss of information on texture and topographical variation may occur as the shadows provided by tangential focal illumination may highlight this. A combination of the two forms of illumination is required.

With diffuse illumination and low magnification attention is spread widely, encompassing the whole field of vision. This is ideal for a general survey of the area. As the beam width narrows and the magnification rises greater detail can be seen, but of a correspondingly more limited area. If we only performed the high-magnification examination we would probably miss something significant while our attention was focused on some tiny detail elsewhere. We should therefore look at the eye in the same way as we would look for a set of keys, with a general reconnaissance of every room before we demolish the sofa.

The following areas should be covered:

1. The external aspects of the lids, looking for signs of inflammation, and swelling.
2. The lashes, looking for signs of:
   (a) **ectropion,** which may be associated with poor drainage
   (b) **entropion** and **trichiasis.**
3. The lid margins, looking for signs of **blepharitis**, which can be associated with changes in both conjunctiva and cornea, and may cause an unstable tear film that could affect contact lens wear. Chronic blepharitis may be encountered as the anterior form, either staphylococcal or seborrhoeic. There is also a posterior type, also known as meibomian gland dysfunction (MGD).

Assessment of the palpebral conjunctiva

To examine the conjunctiva, broad-beam diffuse illumination is used initially, with the emphasis on assessing the degree, depth and location of hyperemia. This may then be followed by more detailed examination using focal illumination. Dyes and stains, and filters may be used to reveal areas of damage.

Severity may be indicated using a grading scale. There are several published grading systems but correlation between them is a little hit and miss and none is accepted universally. The authors tend to favor a simple intuitive scale for all observations as it saves time trying to fit the observation to the photographs or diagrams used in the published versions. If I were a patient, I am not sure I would be very impressed if my practitioner was constantly referring to charts. The intuitive scale used is similar to the one described by Woods (1989) (Table 1.1).

If the observations do not quite fit the gradings we can use plus and minus increments to convert the scale into a nine-point one, which should be sensitive enough for even the most precise observer.

The **distribution of hyperemia** is best recorded as a diagram. Distribution is important. A discrete leash of dilated blood vessels on the bulbar conjunctiva may point to a phlycten. Interpalpebral redness may be associated with drying or with a hypersensitivity reaction to an airborne irritant. Where the hyperemia is greater under one or both lids, we may be dealing with "innocent bystander" (secondary hypersensitivity) reactions from inflamed palpebral conjunctiva.

The **depth of hyperemia** is important in differentiating mere conjunctivitis from episcleritis, scleritis and uveitis, and grading is useful. The injection associated with conjunctivitis tends to be bright red and greatest towards the fornices. Going deeper, the hyperemia associated with episcleritis tends to be salmon-pink and wedge-shaped, with the apex towards the limbus owing to the radial arrangement of the vessels, though the 20% who have the nodular form will show a more circumscribed area of

Table 1.1 **Grading scale for assessment of the palpebral conjunctiva**

Grade	Appearance	Significance
0	Normal	None
1	Slight	Note but no action
2	Moderate	May require action
3	Severe	Requires action
4	Very severe	Refer for medical intervention

redness. Scleritis produces a purplish hue which is diffuse and present all the way to the fornices. Uveitis itself produces deep injection that is most intense around the limbus.

Assessment of the bulbar conjunctiva

In general, the examination of the bulbar conjunctiva will proceed in three sweeps, taking in the upper, middle and lower thirds, with the lids pulled back to see what lies below. In order to view the palpebral conjunctiva, the lids must be everted. Candidates taking professional exams invariably seem to use cotton swabs/buds for this purpose, but with practice many patients can be everted using the fingers alone, and the ubiquitous cotton swab is not an ideal tool for the purpose anyway. The end tends to be too bulbous, and teasing out the fibers will often result in a more useful implement, being easier to insert behind the tarsal margin. The following should be noted:

1. The pattern of any hyperemia, particularly if contact lens-related papillary conjunctivitis (CLPC) is suspected, as it tends to favor the upper lid.
2. Concretions, which appear as discrete yellowish dots. These are of little significance unless they break through to the surface, in which case they are easily removed medically, using a needle.
3. Follicles and papillae seen with diffuse white light initially to look for hyperemia, then focal illumination, directed tangentially, is useful to show the texture as the shadows will be more obvious. With fluorescein instilled, surface texture is enhanced as the dye collects in the channels between the swellings (Figure 1.1).
   (a) **Follicles** are lymphatic in origin, so they themselves are avascular. They appear as multiple discrete, slightly elevated bodies that are translucent and shaped rather like a rice grain (arborio rather than basmati). As they grow they displace the conjunctival vessels, so they can appear with a vascular capsule surrounding the base. They are generally small, but can measure up to 5 mm in severe or unusually prolonged disease.

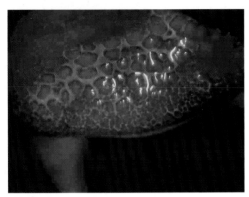

Figure 1.1
Fluorescein emphasizes elevations on the palpebral surface

(b) **Papillae** have their origin in the palpebral conjunctival tissue and consist of a central vascular tuft surrounded by a diffuse infiltrate largely composed of white blood cells. They can only occur where the conjunctival epithelium is attached to the underlying levels by fibrous septa. This restricts them to the palpebral conjunctiva and limbal area. Giant papillae occur when these septa are ruptured.

The tear film

A series of observations can be made of the tear film:

1. **Tear prism height** may be observed by observing the tear prism in section. The normal tear prism is about 0.2–0.4 mm in height, and it appears convex in section. A scanty tear film will have a low meniscus (less than 0.2 mm), which will appear concave. Irregularity of the prism along the lid edge suggests a poor tear film.
2. **Dust particles and bubbles** can be observed within the lower rivus under high magnification. In the normal tear film, particles on the surface move more slowly than deeper ones, due to surface tension. If the movement of particles is too fast, a thin, watery tear film is indicated. Immobile particles reveal excessive viscosity in the tear film.

3. The **tear break-up time (TBUT)** may be assessed by instilling fluorescein then waiting for a few seconds for the tear film to stabilize while the patient blinks. The eye is illuminated with a broad beam and the cobalt blue filter. The patient is then instructed not to blink, and the time noted for dark spots or streaks to appear in the tear layer as it breaks up. Normally this would take 15–20 seconds, and anything below 10 seconds is probably abnormal. Where the same area consistently breaks up rapidly, this is due to a surface irregularity rather than dry eye.

4. **Non-invasive tear break-up time (NIBUT)** can be measured by observing keratometer mires, or a Keeler Tearscope-Plus may be used to project a grid pattern onto the eye's surface, which is then observed for distortion as the tear film breaks. Typical NIBUT time for normal patients is around 40 seconds by this method.

5. **The Tearscope** can also be used to observe interference patterns in the tear film, allowing an estimate of the tear thickness to be made. If a Tearscope is not available, some idea of the quality of the tears may be obtained if the first Purkinje image of the slit beam is observed, especially if the illumination is reduced and the beam narrowed. Colored fringes around the Purkinje image, seen in conjunction with an irregular tear prism, strongly suggest a poor tear film (Figure 1.2).

6. **Mucous strands and debris** in the tears can be an early sign of dry eye. This occurs as the mucin layer becomes contaminated with lipid as the tear film breaks up. Mucin may also combine with cellular debris in more severe cases and form filaments, which are attached to the epithelial surface and move with each blink. Mucous plaques, whitish-gray translucent lesions of varying shape, may appear in concert with the filaments. Fluorescein will reveal punctate epitheliopathy, either in the inferior portion of the cornea or in the interpalpebral area.

7. Damage may also be revealed by the use of **rose bengal** stain. This stains dead and devitalized cells and mucus red. Typically, dry-eye patients show staining of the interpalpebral bulbar conjunctiva, with two triangular areas of stain either side of

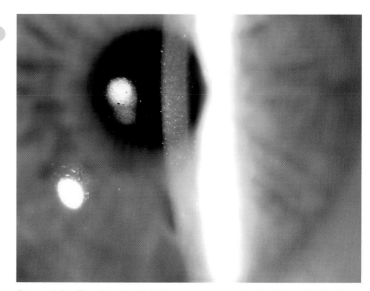

Figure 1.2 The first Purkinje image may reveal color fringes indicative of an unstable lipid layer

the cornea with their apices towards the inner and outer canthi. Mucous strands, filaments and plaques will also show up better with rose bengal. The drawback to rose bengal is that it is a considerable ocular irritant, and, as luck would have it, this quality is rather worse in dry-eye patients. Lissamine green SF (wool green, light green SF), which stains dead cells and mucus blue–green and is less of an irritant, appeared in the 1960s as an alternative to rose bengal. It is available in the USA as impregnated strips but is at present unavailable commercially in the UK.

General examination of the cornea

The magnification used for the initial examination of the cornea is important. If this is set low, the whole cornea (indeed, half of the patient's face) can be covered in one sweep. Unfortunately very little of clinical significance can be detected. This may be initially reassuring for both patient and practitioner, but the longer-term consequences for both are unattractive. An initial examination at too high a magnification would take rather a long time, even assuming that the full consciousness of both parties can be maintained for the duration. It is also far too easy to become lost if the field of vision is too small to contain reference points to navigate by. Therefore, initially, the cornea is examined with medium magnification, set so that the whole cornea may be seen in three horizontal sweeps. If an anomaly is detected the magnification can be increased to allow a closer look.

This angle between the slit beam and the visual axis of the microscope is important for a number of reasons. It allows deeper structures to be observed without an overlay of reflected light from more superficial structures, and this enhances clarity considerably. The wider the slit beam, the greater becomes the angle between the beam and the microscope required to achieve this separation. Another happy consequence of an angled beam is that it is possible to view the cornea by direct, indirect and retro-illumination simultaneously (Figure 1.3).

The area of cornea where the beam strikes is directly illuminated, and, if the observer looks to either side of this bright area, the cornea may be seen in indirect illumination. Opacities will scatter light and be seen as light areas against a dark background (Figure 1.4). A dark background is essential for this, so the room lighting should be off.

To the opposite side of that from which the beam is directed will be an area of cornea which is backlit by reflected light from the iris. Opacities here will appear in silhouette, dark against a light background (Figure 1.5).

For the initial examination of the cornea the beam width should be set at about 2 mm or so, which will illuminate a thick slice of the cornea termed a **parallelepiped**. An angle of 45–60° between beam and microscope allows some appreciation of depth since the edge of the parallelepiped on the opposite side to that from which the light is coming is, in effect, an optical section of sorts (Figure 1.6).

The beam is swept slowly from the limbus to the central cornea. Most authorities recommend that the illumination is from

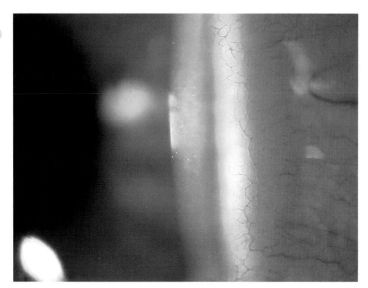

Figure 1.3 Simultaneous direct, indirect and retro-illuminations

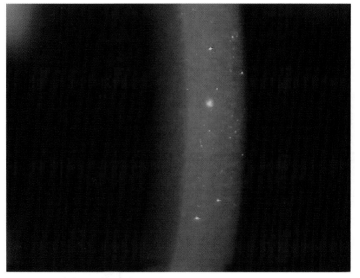

Figure 1.4 Direct illumination shows opacities as light areas

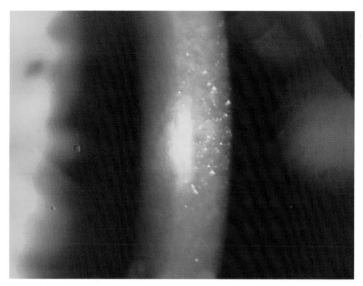

Figure 1.5 Retro-illumination shows opacities in silhouette

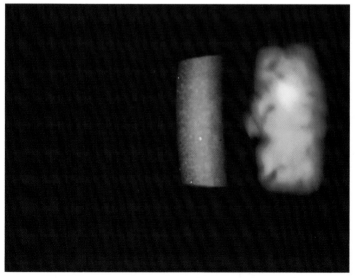

Figure 1.6 A parallelepiped

the same side as the hemicornea being examined, i.e. when observing the cornea to the left of the midline the lamp is positioned to the left of the microscope, the illumination system being swung round to the other side as the midline is crossed. However, the authors prefer to sweep from limbus to limbus with the illumination from each side in turn. Light bounced from the iris can then be employed to retro-illuminate the limbal arcades on the "wrong" side.

When the beam is directed to the limbus, it may be worth widening the beam momentarily and observing the cornea with the naked eye, particularly if the patient already wears polymethyl methacrylate (PMMA) or low Dk RGPs. The light under these circumstances is internally reflected within the cornea and a bright glow may be seen around the limbus. Dense central edema will cause the internally reflected light to scatter and produce a gray glow seen against the dark pupil area. It is possible to decouple the instrument in order to view the cornea through the microscope, but since the demise of PMMA (see Chapter 2) this is rarely necessary. The technique is referred to as **sclerotic scatter**, and it is really only a version of indirect illumination. Sclerotic scatter can also be useful when observing the limbal arcades. A 1–2 mm angled beam is directed at the sclera immediately adjacent to the limbus. The microscope remains coupled, but attention is directed to the limbus and the area of the cornea immediately inside it. The limbal arcades can be seen illuminated partly by internally reflected light and partly by light reflected back off the iris.

The sweeps are performed with the patient looking slightly down, looking level and looking slightly up, and new users should be careful to remember all three. For some reason, optometry students have the unfortunate habit of forgetting to look at the upper cornea, particularly if they look at the other parts first and detect any anomalies. The area of cornea under the lid is particularly likely to develop anomalies due to hypoxia, since oxygen levels are generally lower under the lid, and may also show "innocent bystander" effects such as the keratitis associated with CLPC, due to close proximity to the lid. For this reason it is a good idea to get into the habit of viewing the upper cornea

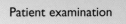

first every time. At this stage we are essentially looking for opacities:

1. Infiltrates indicate active or recently active inflammation. Some patients show one or more small discrete infiltrates distributed at random. These are rarely significant and are probably related to environmental pollution but are worth noting, if only to save wasting time on them later.
2. Scars indicate past inflammation which may be related to infection.

Specific examination of the cornea

Examination at high magnification may be undertaken either because general examination has detected an anomaly or because the history or symptoms of the patient suggest that a specific anomaly may be present. For example, an existing soft contact lens wearer might have microcysts or neovascularization. However, even patients with no history of contact lens wear may have microcysts or vacuoles, and it is important to note their presence in order to differentiate them from those caused by lenses.

Any anomaly of the cornea should be recorded in detail:

1. **Where is it?** Accurate recording of the distance from the limbus (or center) and the clock position makes it easier to find the anomaly again. The estimation of distances when the eye is under magnification is a challenge to the inexperienced microscopist, and this can cause unnecessary alarm when applied to suspect neovascularization, for example. Some slit-lamp microscopes have a graticule eyepiece, which can be useful when making quantitative observations. However, some observers (including the authors) find the graticule distracting. Reasonable estimates of dimensions may be made with a little practice by comparing the size of the object of attention with a known dimension. The visible diameter of the cornea is 11–12 mm, and the amount by which a normal soft lens exceeds it is about a millimeter all round. Alternatively, one can

always hold a millimeter rule close to the anomaly (but be careful!).

2. **How big and how many?** With a wide beam and lowish magnification, the size of a large opacity, or the number of multiple opacities, may be determined. Large single opacities may be associated with bacterial infection or the later stages of herpetic ulceration, whereas multiple smaller ones may be caused by a non-microbial agent or by a viral or protozoan infection.

3. **Color and density** are best assessed with direct illumination. Though most corneal lesions tend towards the monochrome, a hemorrhage within the cornea would give rise to a red lesion and a rust stain might betray a ferrous foreign body. Some of the less dense lesions are more or less invisible under direct illumination and may only appear under indirect or retro-illumination, the classic example being ghost vessels (see below). Oscillation of the beam so that the type of illumination alternates may be useful, and can be achieved either by use of the joystick or by decoupling the instrument and swinging the illumination system independently.

4. The **depth** of an infiltrate or scar tends to correlate with the seriousness of its cause. Intraepithelial infiltrates are usually a response to a non-microbial trigger, though this may include bacterial exotoxins. The deeper, subepithelial and stromal infiltrates are more likely to be associated with infection, and may lead to scarring. Depth perception through a biomicroscope is a result of a composite impression from a series of observations and improves with practice. Experienced microscopists often appear to fidget with both the illuminator and the microscope, seemingly at random to the casual observer. However, valuable information can be gleaned from these maneuvers, even though much of it may be subliminal to the microscopist.

(a) Varying the position of the light source will affect the degree to which the scattered light from layers near to the surface will interfere with the clear resolution of objects in the deeper layers. Parallax between the object and the leading edge of the parallelepiped is also induced.

(b) Swinging the microscope will also create parallax between structures at different levels (see below).

(c) The microscope allows binocular fixation, so stereopsis may be used provided the array is sufficiently detailed.

(d) Not all layers of the cornea will be in focus at the same time, particularly at high magnification when the depth of focus is small.

(e) By far the best way to determine the depth of a lesion within the cornea is to narrow the beam and observe the resultant thin optical section through a microscope set at a considerable angle to the illuminating system.

(f) The other very useful property of a thin section is that elevations and depressions in an interface or surface will cause the beam to deviate. Elevations move the beam towards the side that the light beam is coming from; depressions bend it away from the source. Where the cornea is perforated there will be a gap in the corneal section. To make the most of this effect an angled beam is essential.

Blue light examination of the cornea

The use of fluorescein to examine epithelial integrity is a vital part of every corneal examination, and there is no valid reason not to do it. If there is concern that a patient's soft lenses will be discolored the patient can always be given a daily lens to wear home. Fluorescein colors the tear film rather than staining the tissue. Normally the lipid membranes of the epithelial cells prevent ingress of the substance, but if this is breached by trauma or disease the tear layer gains access to deeper layers. The absorption spectrum and the degree of fluorescence depend on pH peaking at 8. The underlying tissues, because they have a different pH to the surface, will fluoresce more, so the defect is shown up as a green area. In the deeper layers, the fluorescein does diffuse sideways, tending to exaggerate the area of the lesion, and this spread of fluorescein in the stroma may be a useful clue in itself when evaluating epithelial defects. When using the cobalt filter it should be remembered that considerable light has been filtered out, and the rheostat adjusted to give a bright beam. Contrast may be considerably enhanced by the use of a yellow filter (Wratten no. 12 or no. 15) to eliminate reflected blue light from the cornea (Figure 1.7) though recently a lemon yellow filter has been found to be even more effective.

Magnification should also be appropriate. Fine punctate staining cannot be detected at low magnification and may be significant. Fluorescein in the tear film may make corneal staining more difficult to see. It helps if the instillation is frugal, as fluorescein will dye the patient's face or clothing at least as well as their corneas. A short delay (a minute or two) between instillation and observation is useful, to allow the tears to dilute the fluorescein. Fluorescein staining is best recorded as a diagram to illustrate its distribution, along with a grading to indicate severity.

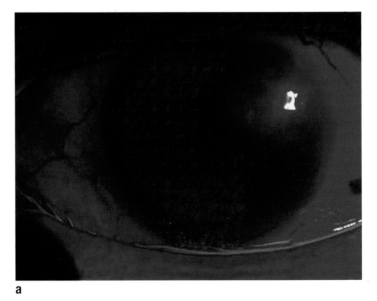

a

Figure 1.7 The absorption of blue reflected light (a) and with a yellow filter (b) (courtesy of Topcon)

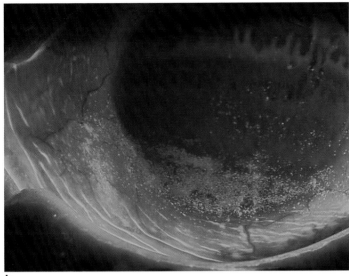

b

Figure 1.7   *Continued.*

References

Tomlinson A, Pearce EI, Simmons PA, Blades K (2001) Effects of oral contraceptives on tear physiology. *Ophthalmic Physiol. Opt.* **21**:9–16.
O'Donnell C, Efron N, Boulton AJM (2001) A prospective study of contact lens wear in diabetes mellitus. *Ophthalmic Physiol. Opt.* **21**(2):127–38.
Woods R (1989) Quantitative slit lamp observations in contact lens practice. *J. Brit. Contact Lens Assoc.*, Scientific Meetings:42–45.

2
Rigid lens materials

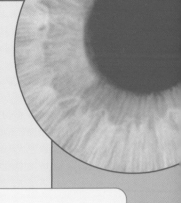

Introduction

An understanding of the material that an RGP lens is manufactured from is vital these days, as it can dramatically affect the on-eye performance of the lens. A brief glance at the manual of the Association of Contact Lens Manufacturers (ACLM) reveals a bewildering list of different lenses and it is easy to wonder where to begin. However, it is not quite as complex as it looks. For a start, there are only a limited number of materials produced, and most contact lens suppliers source their material from the same few places. If you look at the actual material in the ACLM manual the number of choices starts to come down, as one manufacturer's range will be pretty similar to another's, at least for the bread-and-butter lenses. Secondly, many of the materials on offer are obsolete and only still offered because practitioners still order them. Better options are arriving on the market at regular intervals and the manufacturers are rarely reticent about announcing their arrival both in the professional journals and via their own publicity mechanisms. A brief tour through the materials available today will also place the materials in their historical context.

PMMA, TPX and CAB

The ancestor of all rigid gas-permeable lenses emerged in 1947, a lens with a single back surface curve made of polymethyl methacrylate (PMMA). As befits a parent, it had half of the characteristics that we would associate with its RGP offspring in that it was rigid, but not permeable to oxygen. It had very good optical clarity, dimensional stability and durability and it wetted quite well. It was easy to use in manufacturing and was used to make a diverse range of products, from toothbrush handles to geometry sets.

By the 1960s, research and clinical experience had shown that PMMA lenses were not able to deliver adequate levels of oxygen to the cornea to ensure long-term corneal health, and the search was on to find a permeable alternative. In addition, it was believed at the time that a more flexible material than PMMA would improve lens comfort. Most thermoplastics are both more permeable and more flexible than PMMA. Materials such as cellulose acetate butyrate (CAB) and poly4-methyl pentylene (TPX) were initially promising but lacked dimensional stability. This would not have been a major problem, but neither material transmitted a great deal of oxygen, and the emergence of the silicone acrylates soon eclipsed them.

Silicone acrylates

Silicone rubber has an oxygen permeability approximately 100× that of PMMA. However, it shares with all its fellow elastomers a surface which is inherently hydrophobic. Surface treatments have never properly overcome this, and the treated surfaces have a nasty habit of reverting to their previous state. Secondly, the rapid elastic recovery of the materials makes the lens "grab" the cornea after a blink, rather like a suction cup. This can damage the cornea mechanically and cause the lens to bind. There are stories that some of the early clinical trials ended with lenses having to be removed under anesthetic. From this less than promising start it is perhaps no surprise that no true elastomer has been used successfully commercially as a contact lens material.

It would therefore seem an obvious step to combine the virtues of PMMA with the permeability of silicone rubber. The problem is that the two have inherently incompatible chemistries associated with their molecular structure. The solution was to attach units of silicone rubber to a modified methyl methacrylate molecule, which produced the siloxymethacrylate monomer generally known as TRIS.

The first well known silicone acrylate (SA) lens to emerge was Polycon (Wesley-Jessen) which arrived in the late 1970s. By modern standards it had a very low Dk of 8, so it had to be made very thin, which made it rather flexible. It was generally seen as a "lid attachment" fit, large and flat. In the 1980s, the silicone content was increased as manufacturers engaged in the "great Dk race." Paraperm (Paragon Vision) and Boston (Bausch and Lomb) emerged at this time. However, increased permeability was obtained at the cost of increased scratching and surface deposition. Dimensional stability also suffered, with minus lenses flattening and plus ones steepening. Crazing of the lens surface was also reported, though this may have been as much due to manufacturing methods as to the material itself, as too-rapid polishing can heat up the lens surface and produce this effect. The surface of a SA lens is largely hydrophobic, so hydrophilic components such as methacrylic acid were added to improve wetting. The inherent flexibility of lenses with a high silicone rubber content can cause suction on the cornea and there can be adherence and corneal damage.

Fluorosilicone acrylates (FSAs)

The addition of fluorine to the mix was the way to address some of the problems associated with SAs. Fluorine is fairly oxygen permeable, though not as permeable as silicone. Unlike silicone, which relies on diffusion for oxygen transmission, fluorinated polymers allow solubility, soaking up oxygen molecules like a sponge. FSAs are harder than SAs, allowing a better polish. Fluorine also has a low coefficient of friction and low surface tension, which prevents deposits adhering to the lens. After all, a fluoro-polymer related to those used in contact lenses is Teflon, used in non-stick cookware. FSAs are relatively resistant to protein deposition and the weekly enzyme cleaning needed with SAs is rarely needed. Lipid deposits do occur, and certain solutions such as Boston Advance (Bausch and Lomb) are formulated to be effective against lipid deposits on FSA lenses. Mucus also has an affinity to fluorine and a layer of tear film mucin (glycocalyx) forms round the lens. This reduces dehydration and improves tear break-up time, and may allow shorter adaptation times. The only slight problem is that, for a given Dk, FSA lenses tend to flex more than lenses that contain no fluorine. FSAs are the first choice lenses for many practitioners and examples include Fluoroperm (Paragon Vision Sciences), Boston Equalens and RXD.

Fluorocarbons

These are composed of fluorine and methyl methacrylate, with n-vinyl pyrrolidone added to improve wetting. High fluorine contact will produce a lens with reasonably high oxygen permeability (Dk/t about 100), wettable and protein resistant, but very flexible. The Advent (Ocular Sciences) lens is of this type.

Hyperpurified delivery system (HDS)

This is spin-off of NASA's space shuttle research. Hyperpurified silicone is used, which allows a lens of higher permeability and surface wetting without sacrificing lens stability or ease of manufacture. HDS (Paragon Vision Sciences) is available in versions with Dks of 40 and 100 ISO barrers units.

Boston EO

Boston EO (Bausch and Lomb) uses a polymer backbone known as Aerocor which allows oxygen permeability independent of silicone, and the replacement of impermeable PMMA with "bulky esters." This allows the reduction in silicone content by up to 50%, resulting in better wetting while improving dimensional stability. The Dk is 82.

High index

One of the drawbacks to increased oxygen permeability is that refractive index has tended to drop, so lenses must be made thicker. With high powered lenses this can be a problem and a lens with a refractive index of 1.513 as opposed to the more usual 1.455 will allow lenses of about 15% less mass while maintaining oxygen delivery to the eye.

Surface treated lenses

Surface treatment may be achieved by bombarding the surface with oxygen ions in a plasma chamber, as in the case of various Menicon RGP materials. It can also be done by a process called graft polymerization, where a more hydrophilic polymer coating is applied, as in the Millennium (Vista Optics) lens. The result of either is a more comfortable lens that will wet more easily. However, a heavy-handed approach to cleaning (not a common problem admittedly) could wear the surface in time, adversely affecting the lens performance. It is possible that in time surface treatments will emerge with other desirable characteristics, such as bacteriostatic properties.

"Hybrid" lenses

Hybrid FS and Hybrid FS Plus (Contamac) are made of an innovative mixture of FSA and a hydrophilic component, whose unhydrated form is distributed throughout the lens matrix. In contact with solution, the surface hydrophilic molecules bind with the solution, creating an extremely wettable surface. The "FS" part of the name refers to this fluid surface technology. Because the hydrophilic component is not confined to the surface, wearing out is not an issue. There are obvious applications for this type of lens in patients with less than ideal tear films but they may well become first choice lenses in time as they seem to offer no obvious drawbacks.

Classification of RGP materials

EN ISO 11539: 1999 sets out the international standard method for the classification of contact lens materials and as a published European Standard (EN) it has the status of a British Standard and supersedes those BS classifications in previous use. Each material is classified by a six-part code as shown in Table 2.1.

Table 2.1 **Classification code for contact lens materials**

Prefix	This is administered by USAN (United States Adopted Names) and is optional outside the USA. The prefix denotes the polymer used
Stem	This is always focon for rigid lenses, filcon for soft lenses
Series suffix	Administered by USAN. A indicates the original formulation, B the second version, C the third, etc.
Group suffix	I Does not contain silicon or fluorine
	II Contains silicon but not fluorine
	III Contains both silicon and fluorine
	IV Contains fluorine but no silicon
Dk range	A numerical code which identifies the permeability in ranges. The units are cm^2/s $[mlO_2 / (ml.hPa)]$
Modification code	A lower case letter denoting that the surface has been modified and has different characteristics to the bulk material

The Dk range codes are shown in Table 2.2 (after ACLM, 2006).

As an example, let us consider the material Parflufocon B III 3. Its classification says that it consists of a polymer with the USAN prefix Parflu, and that it is a rigid lens material (focon). The suffix B indicates that is the second generation of this polymer and III that it contains both silicon and fluorine. The suffix 3 shows its Dk to be between 31 and 60. It is in fact the classification for Paragon HDS, mentioned above. Boston IV, a silicone acrylate with a Dk of 14, is classified as Itafocon B II 1.

In the past, published information on lens characteristics has tended to be contradictory and confusing. Dks can be measured by a number of methods and manufacturers were fond of quoting the highest figure found for their own lenses by any method. They

Table 2.2   **Contact lens DK range codes**

Group code	Dk range	Examples
1	1–15	Boston ES/IV
2	16–30	Quantum 1
3	31–60	Boston EO/7/Equalens
		Paragon HDS
4	61–100	Boston XO
		Quantum 2
		Paragon HDS 100
5	101–150	Europerm 120
		CIBA Aquila
6	151–200	Flouroperm 151
7	200–250	Menicon Z
Higher codes can be added in bands of 50		

tended to develop a more conservative approach when quoting the Dk of a rival's lenses. This is basic marketing practice but does cause confusion among practitioners and less qualified internet browsers. The ISO classification specifies methods to be used for RGP and soft lenses and the ACLM manual lists Dks in "New Fatt units" which give Dk values approximately 75% of those previously specified. When comparing lenses, make sure that you are comparing like with like, as there is still a bit of creative classification encountered from time to time.

Planned replacement

One of the perceived benefits of rigid lenses is that they have a greater lifespan than soft lenses, and many patients keep the same lenses for several years. In the days of PMMA, lenses would last for years and could be repolished easily to restore them to working order. However, modern high Dk materials do not last as long. Guillon et al (1995) found a measurable decrease in surface wettability after 6 months. Woods and Efron (1996) found that planned replacement of the lenses reduced surface scratching, drying and deposition as well as mucous coating. Additionally, corneal staining, limbal hyperemia and tarsal conjunctival changes might be reduced.

Over time the lenses become gradually less comfortable and the vision may decline gradually. Surface deposition will increase the chances of an immunological reaction. Often these changes are nearly imperceptible, and the patient is surprised how well a new lens performs in comparison with the old one. With modern materials, repolishing is rarely a practical proposition. They are constructed to be as thin as possible to begin with, and some are surface-treated. Furthermore, over-polishing can render the surface hydrophobic.

Planned replacement of the lenses is therefore a useful strategy. The published evidence suggests that the optimum replacement interval might be less than 6 months, but given the cost of manufacturing rigid lenses, 6 months or 12 months is a more practical proposition. In 2003 about half of all RGP lenses in the UK were replaced annually. For extended wear, 3–6 months might be a good idea, as lenses over 6 months old have been found to be more likely to bind.

References

ACLM (2006) Contact Lens Year Book. Association of Contact Lens Manufacturers. Available online at: http://www.aclm.org.uk/.

Guillon M, Guillon JP, Shah D et al. (1995) In vivo wettability of high Dk RGP materials. *J. Br. Contact Lens Assoc.* **18**:9–15.

Woods CA, Efron N (1996) Regular replacement of daily wear rigid gas permeable contact lenses. *J. Br. Contact Lens Assoc.* **19**:83–9.

3
Measurements and initial lens selection

Once we have decided on a material and on the replacement intervals we need to make an initial selection of lens parameters, whether we are going to order a lens empirically or make use of a trial set. Empirical ordering makes this selection rather more critical, as mistakes at this stage can result in patient disappointment when they turn up to find that the lenses you ordered for them have a nasty habit of falling out or that the vision is somewhat blurred. If the next pair is also going to take several days to come through, you might find the patient wandering off to pastures new. However, most of the lenses ordered empirically are quite successful provided care is taken in their selection.

Initial measurements

There are a number of measurements that students of optometry are usually trained to perform, and it is worth considering what they contribute to the selection process for RGP lenses.

The horizontal visible iris diameter (HVID) is usually measured with a ruler (Figure 3.1) but greater accuracy can be achieved by using a measuring graticule on a slit-lamp, thus eliminating parallax errors.

However, even the cruder version is probably more measurement than we really need. Textbooks often say that the total diameter (TD) of the lens should be 1.50–2.00 mm less than the HVID, without saying why, and every year students of optometry solemnly take HVIDs, knock off 2 mm, come up with total diameters to three decimal places and wonder what their supervisors find so amusing. The fact is that all "system" lenses and most custom ones have total diameters between 8.5 and 10.00 mm, which is going to be 1.50–2.0 mm below the normal range of HVIDs anyway, and selection of the total diameter has more to do with interaction of the lens with the eyelids than with corneal diameter. The only RGP patients for whom HVID is worth recording are those with abnormally large or small ones (megalo- and micro-corneal subjects).

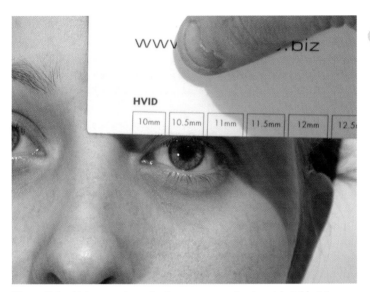

Figure 3.1 Using an adapted rule to measure horizontal visible iris diameter

The visible palpebral aperture (VPA) is also measured, and it does at least give some indication as to how small a lens needs to be to be interpalpebral. Experienced practitioners rarely measure the VPA unless it is exceptional, and rather more useful information can be recorded by drawing the position of the lids in relation to the cornea (Figure 3.2).

The position of the upper lid can influence the degree of lid attachment obtainable with a given diameter. The position of the upper lid prior to fitting may also be worth noting because long-term rigid lens wear can induce ptosis. The shape of the lids can influence horizontal centration, particularly if the lids are tight. The lower lids, if particularly low, can be associated with lower corneal drying and with dropping lenses, particularly with prism-ballasted torics and translating multifocals.

The **pupil diameter** is also measured, both in normal ambient conditions and in poor light, usually using a Burton lamp. The idea is to try to prevent "flare" from

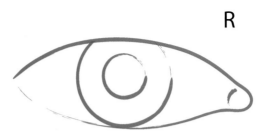

R

Figure 3.2 Example of sketch noting relationship of lids to eye

unwanted reflections from the peripheral curves of the lens by
ensuring the **back optic zone diameter (BOZD)** of the lens
is larger than the pupil. The pupil diameter will be at its largest in
the dark, and the usual method recommended is to measure
this with the room light on and the eye illuminated with a
Burton lamp. However, in anyone with dark irides the process is
one of pure guesswork. For most lenses it is difficult to see how
knowing what the pupil diameter is in "average" light condition
would help much, even assuming there is such a thing as "average"
illumination. There are occasions when fitting multifocals when
this information would be useful, although direct observation
of the lens on the eye is rather more conclusive and patient
satisfaction more relevant. It is also worth considering how
much we are likely to be able to vary the BOZD. Generally the
BOZD is related to the total diameter, and most lenses fall into
the 9.00–9.60 range of diameters. Half a millimeter is not likely
to make a huge difference to flare. The other thing to bear in
mind is that flare is not really much of a problem to most RGP
patients. It's a bit like the scotoma associated with a spectacle
frame. Most people get over it, because they are adaptable. The
ones who do not are rarely entirely happy with any compromise
because they are fundamentally not very adaptable. Life is
probably too short to worry much about flare. If the patient
does worry unduly about it then fit them with a soft lens, or
get a friend to do it.

Selecting the diameters

Clearly, much of the initial measurement with aim of selecting a total diameter is ritual observance rather than actually useful. So how do we decide how big a lens we want, and why? The diameter of the lens influences the degree and type of lid/lens interaction. Smaller, **interpalpebral** lenses rely more on interaction with the cornea to determine their centration but they can be uncomfortable as the edge of the lens may contact the sensitive lid margin during the blink cycle. If we can tuck the edge under the upper lid, away from the margin, the lens is likely to be more comfortable. In addition the lid could hold the lens in position when the eye is open and then move it about a bit during a blink to aid tear circulation. It is possible to rely on lid attachment completely by fitting large flat lenses, though this is not as commonly done now as it once was. On a cornea without a great deal of astigmatism, a larger optic diameter will allow us to spread the weight of the lens and the force of the blink on the lens over a large area. The greater the area of lens in close alignment to the cornea, the greater is the capillary force generated to hold the lens in place. We shouldn't forget also that the larger the optic zone the less flare the patient will see. It is possible to order any BOZD you like, if you are prepared to pay for custom lenses, but unless you leave enough room for the peripheral curves the transition from central to flatter peripheral curves is likely to be too abrupt. This can upset the tear exchange under the lens. For this reason the BOZD is usually about 1.5 mm smaller than the TD.

For all the above reasons, the simple rule when selecting a total diameter is as follows. Pick a big one (9.60 or thereabouts) unless there are good reasons not to. Good reasons include:

1. **Astigmatism**. The larger the TD, the greater will be the difference between the sags in the two principal meridians of the cornea. In other words, if you fit the lens to align with the flatter corneal meridian and the other meridian is appreciably steeper, the lens may be very flat in this meridian, center like

a half-brick, and be a touch uncomfortable. As the degree of corneal astigmatism goes up, the BOZD should come down to allow reasonable alignment in both principal meridians. Once you get to about a diopter of corneal astigmatism, the optic zones on 9.60 diameter lenses start to be a bit large, so it is time to try a 9.30 or 9.00. If the BOZD is small enough, quite large corneal cylinders can be accommodated. Three diopters is usually about the limit, but many practitioners would claim to have overcome more with small (8.00–8.50) diameter lenses. One of the authors did once successfully fit a cornea with 6.00D of corneal astigmatism with an Averlan lens of 7.00 mm diameter. Admittedly the VPA was only 5.00 mm.

2. **Flexure.** RGP lenses are supposed to mask corneal astigmatism due to the tear film between the back surface of the lens and the cornea. Unfortunately modern lenses are made thin to maximize oxygen transmission and this allows a certain amount of flexure. The degree varies with material and lens thickness, but lenses can flex about 30% of the total toricity of the cornea. Flexure creates uncorrected astigmatism in the over-refraction, and if the lens changes shape during the blink cycle because of the lid forces acting upon it, suction can be created under the lens as it returns to shape after a blink. This can affect the epithelium.

3. **Lid interference.** If the lids are tight they may prevent the lens from centering properly. A lens with a total diameter smaller than the VPA may be required to minimize lid interaction with the lens. However, the result may be uncomfortable.

4. **Neovascularization.** Where a former soft lens wearer is being fitted, a smaller lens may avoid the area where new vessel growth has arisen.

5. **Corneal fatigue.** Long-term PMMA and low Dk RGP wearers may experience the "corneal fatigue syndrome" due to chronic hypoxia. One approach to management is to refit with a high Dk material, but with a design similar to the PMMA lens the patient is already wearing. The idea is that once the cornea has settled down the lens will probably still fit well, given that it got the patient this far even with no oxygen transmission. PMMA lenses were generally fitted with

TDs around 9.00, and relatively wide peripheral zones with high axial edge lift (typically 0.12–0.15 mm). The generous peripheral clearance means that the lens is unlikely to develop a sealed edge, even if the cornea flattens during recovery.

The front optic zone diameter (FOZD) of the lens should be at least 0.5 mm bigger than the BOZD. Most lenses are lenticulated to reduce thickness and weight, although it is possible to order non-lenticulated ones. Non-lentics are only really useful as a last resort if the lenses won't center properly. It is also possible to order a negative carrier in order to improve lid attachment. This is usually done on lenses of positive power that tend to drop. A positive carrier, where the edge is tapered, may be used to reduce lid attachment in a high-riding lens.

It is always a good idea to select diameters before thinking about radii. This is because of the shape of the cornea, which is the next thing to discuss.

Keratometry and corneal topography

Keratometry is still the most common measurement of corneal shape performed in optometric practice, and until fairly recently it was usually the only one. The cornea is known not to be spherical but its precise shape has been difficult to pin down. In general it can be described as a prolate ellipse (Guillon and Ho, 1994). That is to say it flattens towards the periphery. The degree of flattening (asphericity) can be expressed in terms of "eccentricity" or as a "shape factor." The average eccentricity for the human cornea is 0.39, which correlates to a shape factor of 0.85. The problem is that it does not always flatten at the same rate, as shape factors vary between +0.50 and −0.10. A negative value indicates a cornea that steepens peripherally, which occurs in about 3% of the population. There is little correlation between the rate of flattening and the values found by keratometry. Two eyes with the same K reading can have widely differing rates of flattening, even in the same individual. The rates may be different horizontally and vertically.

Modern topographical studies have identified five groups:

1. Round (23% symmetrical, v. low astigmatism).
2. Oval (21% asymmetric, v. low astigmatism).
3. Symmetrical bow-tie (17.5% symmetrical astigmatic).
4. Asymmetric bow-tie (32% asymmetric astigmatic).
5. Irregular (7%, no pattern).

The asymmetric groups are interesting, because they have different rates of flattening in the upper and lower areas of the cornea, which can restrict lens movement. The numerous astigmatic bow-tie group have different degrees of toricity in the upper and lower corneas. This is worth remembering next time your lovingly prepared back surface toric won't do the decent thing and center.

There are variations between different ethnic groups. For example, Chinese corneas tend to be steeper and flatten less towards the periphery. There is little correlation between spectacle Rx and shape factor, though high myopes often flatten less than expected, so tend to fit steeper than their Ks would suggest.

To see this in its clinical context, consider the ubiquitous keratometer. It measures the corneal curvature at points about 3 mm apart (it varies with instrument and corneal curvature), either side of the visual axis. If you like, you can measure each eye three times and average the result. Be it one measurement or three, the value obtained tell us very little about the cornea we are going to be fitting, as we know nothing about the shape factor(s). It all sounds a bit of a nightmare, but remember that we have been fitting rigid lenses for years and the "system" lenses available from most manufacturers have undergone a process of evolution. Generally speaking, if you stick to the manufacturer recommendations or simply order on flattest K or thereabouts, the vast majority of lenses turn out to fit quite well. However, be prepared for surprises if ordering lenses empirically from K readings, due to the inherent unpredictability of it all. You should also prepare the patient for this, to avoid looking foolish.

The alternative in recent years has been to use a photokeratoscope, an instrument which can measure the corneal curvature at many points. These instruments can measure shape factors and provide topographical maps. The more sophisticated versions of these now have software that can analyze the data and suggest a suitable lens design, though opinions sometimes vary on the designs suggested. There are also programs that can simulate the likely appearance of a fluorescein pattern a given lens would generate on that cornea, and to experiment with different lens parameters before ordering a real lens. This is fun, and might be very useful on a difficult cornea, but for the majority of cases seen in general optometric practice the words "sledgehammer" and "nut" spring to mind. However, with practice and a tax break we might all be using such instruments to design our lenses one day. There is even some fitting being done using the data from the "wavefront" analysis normally associated with refractive surgery, so it may one day be possible to fit lenses that will give the patient enhanced visual performance.

Choosing the back optic zone radius

The intended relationship between the cornea and the back optic zone of the lens will depend on the fitting philosophy adopted. The lens is held in place on the cornea both by the eyelids and by surface tension, which acts at the lens edge where it is not covered by the lid. If the edge clearance is excessive no meniscus forms and there is no active surface tension. Reduced edge clearance and edge thickness boost surface tension. Broadly speaking, there are two extreme positions that can be adopted.

- Lid attachment ("big and flat"). Here we have a lens of about 9.50 mm diameter, a BOZD of about 8.40 and a back optic zone radius (BOZR) 0.2–0.3 flatter than K. It needs to be this flat with a BOZD this size in order to be flatter than alignment with the cornea. Essentially, the centration and movement of the lens is controlled by the lids, which pass the lens between upper and lower during the blink cycle. Lenses fitted like this do have a habit of riding a little high, especially in the long term, and exposure stain of the lower cornea is common.

● Interpalpebral ("small and steep"). The lens is fitted with a small TD (typically 8.5-ish) and BOZD to minimize lid interference. Generally the BOZR is fitted to give some apical clearance, and this was often done by adding 25–30% of the corneal toricity to the flattest K, a procedure which has unfortunately persisted into "alignment" fitting, where it is inappropriate. Interpalpebral fits are often rather uncomfortable, owing to the interaction of lens edge and lid margins.

Most lenses these days are fitted for an "alignment" fit that is some way between the two extremes. It should be emphasized that there is not just one way of fitting lenses, and the short history of rigid lenses contains examples of very flat and very steep (0.3 mm in the Bayshore method) lenses by modern standards which seemed to work well, at least on some patients. If the standard alignment fit doesn't work another philosophy might, so never be afraid to try something different.

"Alignment" fitting

The idea here is to fit the back optic zone in close alignment with the front surface of the cornea, with a uniform thin tear film between the two. This is a goal rather than something that is actually perfectly realized, but perfect alignment probably wouldn't work very well. The advantages of an alignment fit are as follow:

● The weight of the lens and the force translated through the lens during the blink cycle are spread over the maximum area. If either is too localized, corneal warpage can occur.
● Lens flexure is minimized, which will ensure good visual performance and minimize mechanical stress on the cornea. This is quite an important consideration when using modern high Dk FSAs.

- Provided that the periphery of the lens is also well designed, the thin tear film under the central part of the lens will be easily replenished with oxygen and never become stagnant. Furthermore, a thin tear film will not produce a major "barrier effect," slowing the movement of oxygen through the lens to the cornea. A thicker tear film could produce a situation where the rate of flow of oxygen allowed through the tear film was less than the rate that the lens itself is capable of. Barrier effects reduce the oxygen transmission of all RGPs, especially those with high Dks.

It should be remembered that K readings are taken at points not far away from the corneal apex, whereas we are trying to align an area of cornea over twice as wide. For the majority of patients the spherical curve that will best align with the cornea will be somewhat flatter than K, and the wider the BOZD, the flatter we need to go. In practice, fitting on flattest K seems to work well with conventional designs of 9.00 mm diameter or thereabouts. Once we get up to 9.50 mm we need to go flatter because the average corneal radius is likely to be flatter. On a larger diameter the primary sag of a spherical curve increases, resulting in a steeper-fitting lens. Therefore, if you increase the BOZD by 0.5 mm, you need to flatten the BOZR by 0.05 mm to achieve a "clinically equivalent fit." Most lenses fitted on flattest K are probably a fraction steeper than alignment really, but this seems to work well and may aid centration without seriously compromising in other respects. With an alignment fit, the practice of steepening the BOZR by a proportion of the corneal toricity is inappropriate as any steepening of the fit along the flattest meridian will only serve to push the whole lens further from the cornea, inducing central clearance. It will therefore have no effect on edge stand-off in the steeper meridian, which is the usual intention. It does sometimes help the lens to center, however, if a back surface toric is not an attractive option.

If you are fitting an aspheric design, it is probably best to read the manufacturer's recommendations, as the nominal

BOZR initially selected will be related to the degree of asphericity ("eccentricity" or "shape factor") of the lens design. The principles are similar though.

The periphery

The periphery of the lens may be generated either by working a set (typically three or four) of progressively flatter spherical curves onto the back surface, or as a consequence of using an aspheric curve. In either case, it is worth considering what we have a periphery for. Part of the reason has to do with tear circulation under the lens. If we don't have edge clearance, tear fluid will not be able to get under the lens. This will have two effects. Firstly, the lubricative effect of the tear film will be lost. The lens is then likely to adhere to the epithelium and eventually mechanical damage to this vital layer will occur. Secondly, the oxygen normally carried by the circulating tears will be lost to the cornea under the lens. This is not too important provided the lens is able to transmit sufficient oxygen through its own substance, but for a lens of low transmission tear exchange may be an important source of oxygen delivery. For a PMMA lens it is the only source. Central corneal hypoxia will compromise epithelial integrity further. Clearly, then, we must have enough peripheral clearance to allow adequate tear exchange.

The other reason for peripheral clearance became apparent when silicone acrylate lenses first appeared. Practitioners reasoned that improved oxygen transmission reduced the need for tear exchange, and lenses with very little edge clearance were both more comfortable and tended to center well, owing to the improved tear meniscus around the lens. The downside to all this became apparent when it was time to remove the lenses as a certain amount of edge clearance is needed to allow the eyelids to dislodge the lens. The problem was made slightly worse by the fact that many of the patients being fitted with these lenses were used to PMMA lenses, which needed quite a lot of edge clearance in order to get oxygen to the cornea. Removal techniques made sloppy by loosely fitting lenses (a sharp tap to the back of the head would probably have removed some of the designs then in common use) were severely challenged by the minimal peripheries of the RGPs. A tactical withdrawal to slightly more generous peripheries was undertaken. Modern "system" lenses have peripheries that are worked out by computer to give a smooth progression and where spherical curves are used the transitions between them are polished to "blend" the curves into one continuous surface. They are calculated to work on the majority of patients but if a patient has an unusual corneal shape, too much or too little edge clearance will result. This can be detected once the lens is observed on the eye with fluorescein, and laboratories can increase or decrease the edge lift of the lens produced while keeping the optic zone the same. For a lens ordered empirically, a system lens is usually the best bet, unless you are aware of unusual corneal characteristics.

The terms "edge clearance" and "edge lift" are not interchangeable. Edge clearance refers to the gap between the front surface of the cornea and the back surface of the peripheral curves, and it is edge clearance that is observable

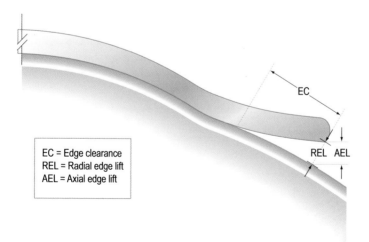

EC

EC = Edge clearance
REL = Radial edge lift
AEL = Axial edge lift

REL   AEL

Figure 3.3 Edge lift and edge clearance

with fluorescein. Edge lift is a geometrical characteristic of the lens itself, and is definable in either axial or radial forms. The difference between them is shown in Figure 3.3.

Edge profile

The shape of the edge is an important determinant of lens comfort, especially in the early stages. Laboratories tend to have their standard designs, but if you find that the lenses coming through are not as comfortable as they should be, you could ask for a different form (or change labs, of course). Generally, for the alignment fit with partial lid attachment it is interaction between the lens edge and the eyelids (rather than the cornea) that seems to determine comfort. Rounding of the anterior rather than the posterior edge seems to be the important factor.

Center thickness

Modern lenses, because of their material properties and thin design, tend to flex, especially in low minus-powered lenses. In general, flexure increases with Dk and with the degree of toricity of the cornea the lens is sitting on. The minimum thickness desirable for a given power is shown in Table 3.1 (after Young 2002). In general, "system" lenses take care of this for you. Once corneal astigmatism gets to about 2.00D a further 0.02 mm is needed, so if you are fitting an astigmatic

Table 3.1 **Minimum center thickness recommended for low minus lenses**

Lens power (D)	Center thickness (mm)
−1.00	0.18
−2.00	0.17
−3.00	0.16
−4.00	0.15
−5.00 and over	0.14

cornea with a spherical lens you might need to order something a bit thicker. This will, of course, compromise the oxygen transmission a little.

Back vertex power

The power of the contact lens required would normally be calculated from the spectacle prescription corrected for vertex distance but must take the power of the tear lens between the contact lens and cornea into consideration. If the lens is in perfect alignment with the central cornea, it follows that the tear lens will have zero dioptric power, and over-refraction is rather a good way to measure the degree of alignment. A lens which is steeper than the cornea will give rise to a tear lens of positive power, and a flat lens will create a negative tear lens. The power of the tear lens can be calculated precisely, but for lenses fitted fairly close to alignment this is unnecessary. A simple rule of thumb exists. For every 0.05 mm that the BOZR is steeper than K, the tear lens power increases by +0.25D. Therefore you must counter this by adding −0.25D to the power of the contact lens. Obviously, if the contact lens is flat by 0.05 mm, an extra −0.25 is added to the power of the tear lens, and the power of the lens ordered must be increased by +0.25D.

Let us consider a simple example. A patient has a spectacle prescription of −5.00DS at a back vertex distance of 10 mm. His K readings are 7.80 mm in all meridians, but we have elected to fit him with a lens with a BOZD of 7.75 mm.

The first step is to adjust the spectacle lens power to account for the fact that the contact lens is sitting on the eye. This can be calculated using the formula

$$L = \frac{Fs}{1 - dFs}$$

where L = power of contact lens
       d = vertex distance of spectacle lens
      Fs = power of spectacle lens.

However, it is much easier to look it up in a table, such as that provided in the ACLM manual. A spectacle lens at 10 mm BVD has an effective power in the corneal plane of −4.75D, so this is the power we need for the contact lens.

The lens is 0.05 mm steeper than K, so the liquid lens will have a power of +0.25D. To counter this we need to add −0.25D to the contact lens power, which takes us back to −5.00D. This is the power we will order.

If we decide that the 7.75 base curve looks a bit steep, we might decide to order a flatter lens next time. Suppose we want to order a BOZR of 7.85 this time. This is 2 × 0.05 mm flatter than the previous lens, so we will create a tear lens with an extra −0.50D. We need to modify the power of the lens we order by +0.50, so we will order −4.50D.

On the other hand, we might not do this, even if it is theoretically indicated, as we also need to consider the inconvenient fact that most of our patients have two eyes. These two eyes usually work together, though sometimes not as well as we might hope.

Binocular considerations

Myopes are likely to be exophoric, particularly at near fixation distances. If they wear their spectacles for near visual tasks, they will benefit from a certain amount of base-in prism at near, as the spectacles will be centered for distance. The loss of this base-in prism may result in decompensation of their near ocular motor balance, variable vision, asthenopic symptoms or even diplopia. In such cases, a slight over-correction of their myopia can sometimes be beneficial, as the extra accommodation stimulated will also induce accommodative convergence. With a normal accommodative convergence/accommodation (AC/A) ratio of around 4 even −0.25D can significantly alter the ocular motor balance without overloading accommodation itself.

Accommodative demand is higher for a myope in contact lenses than it is in spectacles. If the patient habitually reads without spectacles, as many low myopes do, they may initially struggle to cope with the extra accommodative demand that correction of their myopia brings. For these patients, over-correction is not appropriate. Hyperopic patients often find near vision easier with contact lenses, as their accommodative and convergence demands are less. Practitioners should also beware the hyperope with a significant latent element, as their latent element sometimes seems to become manifest shortly after contact lens fitting.

Markings

It used to be common to see lenses marked "R" and "L" and some lenses have the BOZR and TD printed on them as well. This is wonderful when doing aftercare, especially if you didn't fit the patient. However, engravings do tend to assist the formation of deposits and they may weaken a lens mechanically. A spate of RGP lenses splitting in line with the vertical part of the R and L led to many labs adopting a simpler method of discrimination between the two, and most lenses now have only a small dot on one lens, usually the right one. One consequence of this is that many patients, particularly those in early presbyopia, have no idea which lens is which, and may turn up for aftercare appointments with either lens in either eye, or two of the same.

Tints

Some standard lenses come with a handling tint; this is intended to assist the detection of dropped lenses. The concept works well when white bathroom suites are in fashion but less so when the height of lavatorial elegance comes in avocado or tasteful beige. In any case the handling tint is rarely an option and is generally a standard feature of a particular lens. Similarly, many lenses have a UV inhibitor incorporated in the lens polymer and occasionally this is offered as an optional extra. The ACLM manual identifies those lenses with a UV inhibitor. UV filtration may have long-term benefits for ocular health, particularly for those working outside, and for aphakes. On the other hand, you should not attempt to examine the fluorescein pattern of a lens with a UV inhibitor with a Burton lamp. The cobalt blue light on a slit-lamp will give a truer picture on these lenses.

Summary

To order empirically, or to select from a trial set.
  For a cornea with low toricity:

- TD should be large (approx 9.60 mm) unless there are good reasons for it not to be.
- BOZD should be the same as flattest K or slightly flatter. Keratometers vary owing to their different mire separation so get to know your instrument and allow for it.
- Edge lift should be standard unless you know the patient isn't.
- The lens edge needs to be "well rounded" or to have a well rounded front edge.
- Center thickness should be standard unless you are fitting a spherical lens on a cornea with significant astigmatism. In this case add 0.02 to the standard thickness. Manufacturers will usually allow for the flexibility of the lens material in setting their standard thickness.
- Power should be the spectacle correction adjusted for vertex distance and the tear lens, unless you are trying something clever to help ocular motor balance.

References

Guillon M, Ho A (1994) Photokeratoscopy. In *Contact Lens Practice* (ed. Ruben M & Guillon M), pp. 313–57, Chapman and Hall Medical, London.
Young G (2002) Rigid lens design and fitting. In *Contact Lens Practice* (ed. Efron N), pp. 186–202. Butterworth-Heinemann, Oxford.

4
Handling and assessing RGP lenses

The initial selection of the lens might be made from a fitting set or the lens may have been ordered empirically. In either case, we can now insert the lens and assess the fit. This chapter will first consider the handling of RGP lenses, then go on to look at the methods of assessing and recording the fitting characteristics.

Handling RGP lenses

When handling RGP lenses in a clinical setting, a number of factors need to be taken into account. The lens itself is rigid, and it has a rather sharp edge. This gives it the potential to cause an unpleasant injury to the eye. In addition, the patient is likely to be nervous. Research has suggested that many patients are more nervous when having their eyes tested than when visiting the dentist, and the prospect of having something uncomfortable inserted is unlikely to help them relax. It is therefore important that the practitioner be a source of calmness and confidence. This is much easier to achieve if the practitioner is actually calm and confident, and competence in the handling of lenses will soothe the nerves of both parties. The only way to achieve competence is by practice, but a little bit of gamesmanship can go a long way.

When it comes time to insert the lens, don't give the thing too much of a build-up, and a little bit of spin goes a long way. Optometry students often indulge in over-elaborate explanations, accompanied by an expression of strangulated concern suggestive of a digestive disorder. This usually has the opposite effect to that intended, and patient confidence plummets like a stone. A casual, brisk manner work wonders at this point, so get on with it. Avoid words like "hurt" and "pain" and suggest "this might tickle a bit at first, but it will settle down in a couple of minutes." Choice of clothing may have some effect here as well. Pale colors tend to be less threatening than dark ones, particularly if the practitioner is physically imposing.

Before the practitioner touches any part of a patient, including the eyelids, thorough washing of the hands should occur, and the patient should see it happen. This will set a good precedent, reassure the patient about hygiene and hopefully influence his or her own approach to this vital area. If you get into the habit of washing your hands before touching the patient you won't easily forget (though in truth we all have on occasion), even when distracted by a difficult patient or in an unfamiliar consulting room. The hand washing can even be a bit exaggerated, in the same way as looking in the mirror during your driving test.

The conditioning solution should be applied to the lens, but it should be spread over the lens surface rather than used to fill the concave bowl formed by the back surface. This latter procedure just makes the lens heavy and means that it has to be kept concave side up, which makes insertion difficult for those who have no talent as contortionists. The idea is to have enough solution to stick the lens to your finger, but no more. You will then find that you can turn the lens upside down or in any position and it will still stay on your finger until the moment that the surface tension of the tear layer pulls it onto the patient's eye. Most students put the lens on the first finger for their early attempts at lens insertion, but for many practitioners the middle finger is longer. If the lens is placed on the end of this finger the extra length may allow some bending of the finger, which may assist insertion. Whichever finger is used, the lens should be placed on the fingertip, so that the area of contact between the finger and the lens surface is minimal. This makes it easier for the tear film to pull the lens from the finger.

Next, consider how best to approach the eye. There are few things more unnerving for a patient than the sight of a hard thing with sharp edges approaching the eye. Throw in the shaking hands and slow approach of the nervous practitioner and the odds for the lens going in the eye don't look very good. The most likely outcome is for the patient to lose their nerve completely, back away sharply and close their eyes. To prevent this, get the patient to lean the head back against the headrest of the chair. Raise the upper eyelid with the thumb of your free hand. The palm and fingers of the hand are then available to apply gentle but firm pressure should the patient show a tendency to adopt the fetal position. Usually this would be the practitioner's left hand for the patient's right eye. It is worth approaching the eye from a point off the visual axis, so get the patient to look slightly down, preferably at some tangible target such as an electricity outlet on the wall. This will help to keep the eye still, especially if the practitioner keeps saying things like "keep watching the plug…keep watching…keep watching all the time." Moving targets are much harder to catch. With a particularly nervous patient, it might be worth the practitioner standing well to the side or even behind the patient's chair, out of the line of sight. Once the patient is positioned, head on the headrest, looking down, the approach with the lens can proceed.

The lower eyelid should be controlled with one of the fingers of the hand bearing the lens, usually the one next to the one carrying the lens. This steadies the hand and also provides some protection for the cornea if the patient panics and moves forward suddenly. If the hand carrying the lens is braced against the patient, patient, hand and lens all move the same way if the head jerks suddenly.

The approach to the eye should not be too slow. Firstly, it gives the patient more time to lose their nerve, and secondly, both the conditioning solution and the tear film can dry out. If it does dry out the lens tends to stay on the finger of the practitioner. The place to aim for is the upper part of the cornea. This allows an approach oblique to the visual axis and the lens is traveling down when it contacts the eye. Gravity will therefore assist the transfer of the lens from the finger to the cornea. If we were to approach the cornea along the visual axis, it is more likely that we would provoke a defensive lid closure that would be accompanied by Bell's phenomenon, an upward roll of the eye that protects the cornea. The lens is likely to end up on the lower sclera, which, while easily remedied, does tend to upset a nervous patient. There is also the possibility of corneal insult from the lens edge. If the upper cornea is targeted, Bell's phenomenon usually results in the lens landing on the central cornea. If the patient maintains fixation, the lens will contact the tear film and slide gently down upon it to a central position, expelling any air bubbles behind it. Generally the lens should be aimed such that about a quarter of it overlaps the limbus.

Once the contact lens is on the cornea the patient may not be very comfortable, but both the discomfort and the resultant tearing and blepharospasm can be limited if the practitioner keeps talking to the patient. "Rest your head back on the headrest, and look down… That probably feels better already." Suggestion is a powerful tool. Should the patient fail to respond to your blandishments, however, consider the following possibilities:

- There is an air bubble trapped under the lens.
- The lens edge is damaged.
- There is a foreign body under the lens.
- The patient is reacting to the conditioning solution.

As a damage limitation exercise, remove the lens promptly, clean, rinse thoroughly and reinsert, provided the cornea is undamaged. If the lens is still unacceptably uncomfortable, it is probably not an air bubble causing it, so have a look on the slit-lamp.

Some patients show an exaggerated response to foreign body irritation termed an **axon reflex**. This involves efferent fibers of the trigeminal nerve, which cause an inflammatory response. In these cases the eyes go pink, the lids swell up, and the wise practitioner considers whether RGPs are really the best option.

Should the lens settle on the sclera, no attempt should be made to move it onto the cornea. In the grand old days of PMMA lenses, re-centration was a standard maneuver, taught to every optometry student. The reduced edge clearance of modern RGP designs make this a very dubious procedure now, and the likely result is damage to the limbal area from the edge of the lens. Any damage to the cornea increases the risk of serious infection and the limbal area is where the corneal stem cells reside. If the lens gets onto the sclera, take it out and reinsert onto the cornea. You might have to push it round to the temporal sclera first in order to be able to get at it. The "pinch" technique (see page 58) is appropriate here to remove the lens.

This brings us rather conveniently to removal. There are a number of methods, each with advantages and disadvantages.

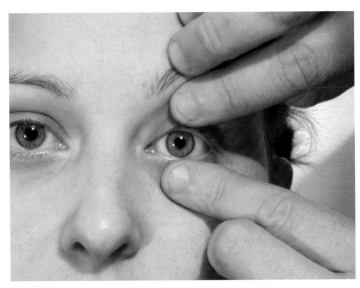

Figure 4.1 Pinch method of removal

The **"pinch" technique** involves controlling the upper and lower lids by placing a finger or thumb on the lid margin of each (Figure 4.1). Starting with the lids parted somewhat wider than the total diameter of the lens, gently bring them together so that the lid margins burrow under the periphery of the lens, thus popping the lens out. If the lids are controlled and positioned correctly, almost no force is required to break the surface tension holding the lens in. The lens should release from the cornea with a gentle "pop" to be collected. If you want to show off, with practice it is often possible to get the lens to settle on a finger or the thumb of the hand controlling the lower lid, which can then be shown to the patient with a bit of a flourish. A cheap and flashy trick undoubtedly, but also a demonstration of skill which can reassure a patient who is nervous that removal might be difficult. The pinch technique is probably the most commonly used technique these days, but it doesn't work on everyone. Some patients respond to touching of their lid margins by going into blepharospasm.

The **"pull and blink"** method used to be the first choice in the days of PMMA lenses, when peripheries had a rather more generous clearance. However, it still works well on many lenses, often in those patients who respond badly to the pinch technique. The method is as follows. The patient fixates an object chosen so that the cornea, and the lens, is positioned between the lids at the point where the interpalpebral distance is at a maximum. The patient is then told to open their eyes as wide as they can. The lids are tensioned by pulling at the outer canthus until the surface tension of the tear film is broken (Figure 4.2). This can be done with a finger, but is usually more easily done with the practitioner's thumb, which has a greater contact area. If the eyes are positioned correctly and the lids tensioned evenly, little force may be required. However, sometimes the tensioning of the lids is insufficient to break the surface tension, and this must be achieved by asking the patient to blink. The lens may be ejected from the eye rather quickly in these circumstances, so be prepared to catch it, unless you would like to spend the next 5 minutes on the consulting room floor looking for the lens. If the blink is rather violent, the patient may hurt the eyelid too.

The **"V" method** is also worth practicing, as it often works on those patients on whom the other two methods don't work. The patient is instructed to look at an object placed so that the eye is abducted. The lids are tensioned by the practitioner using fingers or thumbs so that they form a V, or rather a > with the point at the inner canthus (Figure 4.3). The patient is then instructed to look in towards the nose. The surface tension is broken as the lens catches in the V of the lids, while the eye cornea continues towards the inner canthus.

If all else fails, you can always use a **suction holder**. These handy devices were once found everywhere that contact lenses were fitted, in the days when PMMA and early RGP lenses dominated the market. They seem to have all but disappeared, but if a lens sticks hard on the sclera – as they occasionally do – a suction holder is the tool of choice. It is therefore a good idea to have a supply in the consulting room.

Occasionally a patient will panic and develop blepharospasm. This can make removal of the lens impossible. Fortunately there

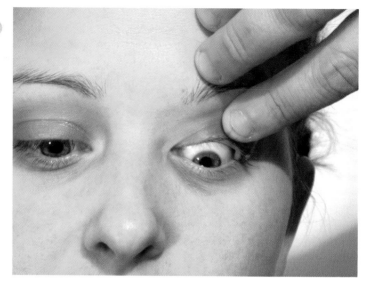

a

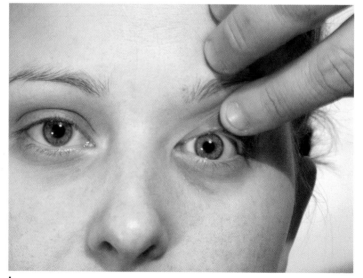

b

Figure 4.2 "Pull and blink" method of removal

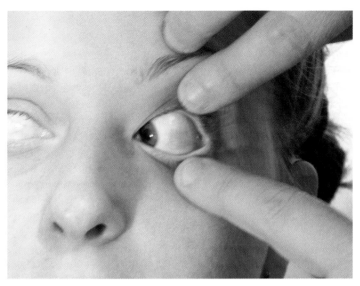

Figure 4.3 "V" method of removal

is a trick which works 99 times out of 100. In a calm, confident tone of voice, address the patient thus: "When I say go, open your mouth as far as you can. GO!" It is almost impossible to close the lids tightly and open the mouth wide at the same time. We are simply not wired up that way. Secondly, the drawing of attention towards the mouth, away from the eye, may also contribute to the effect. Either way, it will usually give you enough time to get the lens out.

Assessing the fit

When assessing the fit of a rigid contact lens, textbooks tell us that we must consider two things:

- The dynamic fit, or how the lens moves and centers on the eye.
- The static fit, or how the back surface of the lens relates to the cornea.

Dynamic fit

On an established wearer the way that the lens moves and
centers is important but on a patient new to rigid lenses the
dynamic fit can be frankly misleading. A tense patient is likely
to have tighter lids than usual. The tear film will be abnormal
both in volume and viscosity as reflex tearing in response to
foreign body overlays the normal background tear secretion.
For this reason some authorities advocate the use of a local
anesthetic during the fitting assessment, though their use may
make the corneal epithelium a little less resilient and the
degree of comfort of the lens cannot be assessed. When lenses
are ordered empirically, it is customary to arrange the time to
teach the patient how to handle the lenses to follow on from
the checking of the fit. Obviously in these circumstances an
anesthetized eye would be dangerous. The tearing may be
exacerbated by white light examination on the slit-lamp. If the
light is unnecessarily bright even more tearing can take place. It
is therefore not surprising that many lenses inserted on patients
unused to RGPs move about somewhat enthusiastically.
Inexperienced practitioners may conclude from this that the
lens is flat fitting.

When observing an RGP lens in these circumstances, it is
important not to get too carried away with fact that the lens is
centering like a half-brick. Provided it stays within the limbus –
and occasionally even if it doesn't at this stage – it will probably
get better once the tear film has normalized. If the lens is
moving vertically with the blink cycle, it is probably not flat. Flat
lenses tend to go sideways, or arc around in a semicircle. Lenses
that decenter horizontally are not always flat. Lid geometry can
sometimes do this, so it is useful to part the lids with the fingers
and see what happens. If the lens does the decent thing and
centers up, there is probably little to be gained by changing the
central fit. Measures must be taken to reduce the influence of
the lids, and that usually involves reducing diameters or
thicknesses.

On an adapted patient, the centration and movement of the
lens is more representative provided we are not attempting

photocoagulation with the slit-lamp. It is a very good idea to use a diffuser when looking at contact lens fit, for both RGP and soft lenses. It spreads the light source, enabling us to see the whole lens evenly illuminated without too much glare for the patient. What we are considering for the most part is how the lens interacts with the lids, because by adjusting the total diameter of the lens, by changing the thickness of the edge or the weight of the lens we can increase or decrease "lid hitch" as required.

Fluorescein assessment of contact lens fit

The relationship between the back surface of the lens and the cornea is investigated by instilling fluorescein into the tear film. This enables us to see a map showing the thickness of the tear layer under the lens. Sodium fluorescein is orange–red in color and, when in dilute concentration in an aqueous solution, is excited by short-wavelength light (peak absorption 485–500 nm) to emit a green light (maximum intensity 525–530 nm). This useful property has been exploited since Obrig first described it in 1938. Before that fluorescein had been in use to investigate corneal lesions for about half a century, using white light! The cobalt blue filter on the slit-lamp causes fluorescence to occur while eliminating wavelengths that have little effect. This reduces veiling glare. In order to improve contrast, a yellow barrier filter (e.g. Wratten no. 12–15) may be placed before the observation system, either built in or attached to the observation system of the instrument or as a cardboard-mounted accessory widely available from contact lens manufacturers. This filters out the reflected blue light from the eye and the background fluorescence of the cornea. Fluorescein has long been used to assess the fitting characteristics of rigid contact lenses, both scleral and corneal. Traditionally this was done using a Burton lamp which employed a pair of "Blacklight Blue" miniature fluorescent tubes. Unfortunately, many RGP materials absorb light in the UV-A band (315–400 nm) with the result that the fluorescein under such a lens will not fluoresce sufficiently to allow accurate estimation of the fit. This is particularly likely with high minus lenses made of the widely used fluorosilicone acrylate materials, where the thickness of the lens in the more peripheral parts of the optic zone can prevent fluorescence, giving the false appearance of a steep fit. The cobalt blue filter of the slit-lamp emits more longer wavelength light, so the fitting characteristics of the lens may be better visualized (Figure 4.4).

The amount of fluorescence emitted by the fluorescein will depend on tear thickness but it is also proportional to concentration, pH and the amount of light used to irradiate it.

Concentration of the fluorescein affects the minimum thickness of tears that will fluoresce. At higher concentrations even very thin layers, such as those found under an aligned lens, will fluoresce, albeit weakly. As the tears dilute the concentration, the same thickness of tears will produce no detectable green fluorescence. It is still the same tear film though. The absence of fluorescence does not necessarily indicate touch. It just means

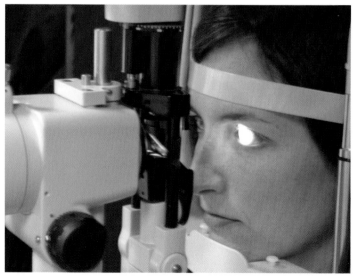

Figure 4.4 Cobalt blue filter (courtesy of Topcon UK)

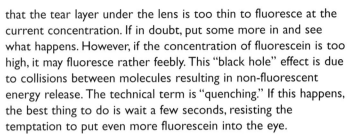

that the tear layer under the lens is too thin to fluoresce at the current concentration. If in doubt, put some more in and see what happens. However, if the concentration of fluorescein is too high, it may fluoresce rather feebly. This "black hole" effect is due to collisions between molecules resulting in non-fluorescent energy release. The technical term is "quenching." If this happens, the best thing to do is wait a few seconds, resisting the temptation to put even more fluorescein into the eye.

The degree of fluorescence is influenced by other factors:

1. The **pH** in the eye and even the pH of the saline used to moisten the Fluoret can affect the fluorescein pattern. The absorption spectrum and the degree of fluorescence depend on pH, peaking when the pH is 8. Buffered saline should be used with fluorescein – or at least always use the same type of saline to ensure consistency.

2. **Illumination** has a major effect on fluorescein patterns. Up to a point (and unless you can smell burning you probably haven't reached it), the more light you put in, the more fluorescence you get back. In order to get a decent fluorescein pattern on most slit-lamps you must turn the rheostat right up. This means that there is enough fluorescence being produced to make a Wratten filter worthwhile. If you use a Wratten with low illumination it won't work, as it, like all filters, subtracts light rather than adds it. The use of the diffusing filter is also recommended, as it allows the whole lens to be illuminated at one time.

Fluorescein is best applied in the form of Fluorets. These impregnated strips circumvent the fact that liquid fluorescein is a splendid culture medium for *Pseudomonas*. On new or nervous patients the moistened strip is best applied to the lower sclera or inner surface of the lower lid, with the patient looking up. That way, if the patient panics and Bell's phenomenon occurs, the cornea is protected. The strip should be touched flat to the sclera or inner surface of the lower lid. Wiping (the "slash" technique) or prodding (the "bayonet") both carry the risk of a paper cut to the eye, which is not a pleasant prospect. When wetting the Fluoret, it is sensible to shake off the excess, unless the patient has specifically requested a tie-dyed shirt in tasteful orange.

Assessment of the fit

The static fit of the lens consists of two elements, which should be considered separately:

- The central zone.
- The periphery.

It is important to consider the position of the lens on the cornea when assessing the fluorescein pattern. The central curves of the lens are usually designed to align with the central area of the cornea, and this can only be assessed if the lens is centered correctly. On new patients, centration may be poor, and the practitioner may have to control the position of the lens with the patient's lids. Failure to do this will result in misinterpretation of the fluorescein pattern. The classic error occurs when a flat lens is allowed to drop so that the central zone of the lens is sitting on a more peripheral part of the cornea. In most patients, the peripheral cornea is rather flatter, and the result can be that pooling of fluorescein will occur under the lens. The lens can then be interpreted as steep. This error can prove expensive.

Central fit and alignment

It is the area under the optic portion of the lens that we should consider first, as it influences centration and movement, flexure and oxygen supply. Usually we are aiming for an "alignment" fit. In other words, we want the tear layer to be uniformly thin over as much of the optic zone as possible. We need, therefore, to consider what this looks like. A thin tear film with a high concentration of fluorescein will have a slight greenish glow. As the fluorescein dilutes, that greenish glow will cease. Provided that the periphery allows efficient tear exchange, an aligned lens should go from high concentration to low rather quickly. Therefore an aligned optic zone will either have a slight greenish glow or none, depending on how much fluorescein you put in and how long ago you put it in. So how do you tell if it is aligned?

The optic zone must be subdivided into two imaginary zones, central and mid-peripheral (Figure 4.5).

To assess the central fit, simply compare the amount of green visible in the two zones:

- If there is more green visible in the central zone than the mid-peripheral one, the lens is steep. As the fit becomes progressively steeper, the diameter of the central green zone contracts, and the contrast between the two zones increases. This is because the tear exchange under the lens is compromised. This also has the effect of prolonging the fluorescein pattern, so a steep lens tends to look the same for minutes on end, rather than the seconds that an aligned pattern may persist.

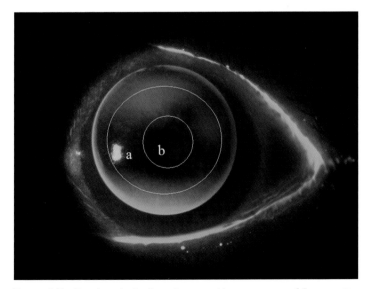

Figure 4.5   Dividing the back optic zone aids assessment of fluorescein distribution under the lens (so in this case, compare the fluorescence in zones a and b)

- If the central area shows no fluorescence but the mid-peripheral zone does, the fit is flat. With increasing flatness, the size of the blue area of "touch" in the center will contract. It should be remembered that "touch" is a misnomer. A thin tear film is present, but not enough to fluoresce detectably.

- An aligned fit should show either a hint of green under the whole optic zone or blue touch. If in doubt, put some more fluorescein in and have another look, when the green glow and its demise should occur in quick succession. However, if the periphery is tight you may not be able to get enough fluorescein under the lens to create a glow even initially. If there is no central glow at any stage, look at the peripheral zone to see if that could be the problem before changing central curves.

The fit should be recorded as aligned, steep or flat with some indication of degree. However, given that half the population have asymmetric corneal curves, something a little more detailed might be useful. Van der Worp and de Brabander (2005) described a system whereby the fluorescein thickness at a number of points on the lens can be graded. A grade of 0 indicates a satisfactory tear thickness, −1 slightly too thin and −2 much too thin. A grade of +1 indicates a tear layer which is slightly too thick, and +2 much too thick. Both central and peripheral fluorescein patterns can be recorded in this way. The system allows greater detail, but it is recorded relative to an anticipated pattern, so it would be worth recording the type of fit against which we are judging the lens (e.g. alignment or interpalpebral) for future reference.

Peripheral fit

The degree of edge clearance that a "system" lens will show depends on the design of the lens and the shape factor of the patient's cornea. It is inadvisable to alter the BOZR and BOZD in order to adjust edge clearance. The parameter to address is **edge lift**, which with modern computer assisted lathes can be easily varied for any given central zone. In general, good peripheral clearance looks like a band of green 0.5–0.75 mm wide under the periphery of the lens (Figure 4.6).

If the green band is too narrow, check that it is actually under the lens, as a sealed periphery may show a thin green band around the edge (Figure 4.7).

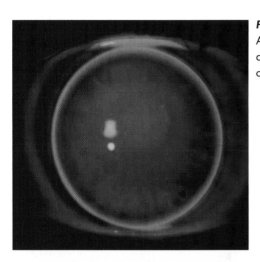

Figure 4.6
Acceptable edge clearance (courtesy of D. Ruston)

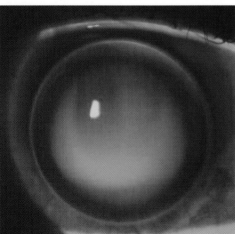

Figure 4.7
Narrow edge clearance zone (courtesy of D. Ruston)

Ideally, the green band should gradually blend into the blue area of "touch." An abrupt change from green to blue indicates a sharp transition. This can compromise tear exchange and cause corneal trauma and the periphery may need "blending" with intermediate curves.

As discussed in the section on lens design, edge clearance is ultimately required to allow tear exchange under the lens and lens removal. The precise physical dimensions required depend on the oxygen transmission and surface characteristics of the material.

It is worth observing the peripheral fit as the lens moves with blinking and excursions of the eye. Dark areas of touch may appear. These may indicate "grounding" of the lens edge, which may result in physical trauma to the cornea. A tight periphery may also restrict movement of the lens. This can cause the lens to decenter, usually downwards. If the lens has a tendency to decenter, look for peripheral touch on the opposite side to the direction that the lens has decentered.

Astigmatic corneas

Spherical lenses on astigmatic corneas produce a characteristic "dumb-bell" shaped fluorescein pattern. For example, let us consider a cornea that shows "with the rule" astigmatism, that is one where the flatter meridian of the cornea and the negative cylinder axis is roughly horizontal. If we fit a spherical optic zone to align with the flatter horizontal meridian, it follows that the lens will be rather flatter than the cornea's steeper vertical meridian (Figure 4.8).

"Against the rule" and obliquely astigmatic corneas will produce similar patterns but at a different orientation. The trick to interpreting these patterns is to identify the principal meridians (not exactly rocket science if you have the spectacle Rx or Ks) and consider the fluorescein distribution along each of them in turn. This avoids the classic student error, where the lens is pronounced flat as opposed to "with the rule aligned," for example, on the evidence of only one meridian.

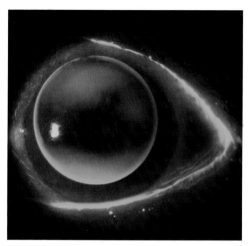

Figure 4.8 Spherical lens on astigmatic cornea (courtesy of D. Ruston)

Further consideration of the fitting of astigmatic corneas will be found in a later chapter.

Troubleshooting

In general, most lenses ordered empirically or selected from a fitting set will not be too far away from optimal, provided the selection is done carefully. This may be news to many students of optometry as one of the most difficult tasks a contact lens examiner faces is to get a student to admit that a selected lens is optimal. However, there are a number of ways in which lenses may misbehave which have simple remedies.

For corneas with low astigmatism

- If the lens decenters horizontally on a near-spherical cornea, part the eyelids to check if the lids are causing this. If they are, a smaller, interpalpebral lens may help, though discomfort may be an issue. If the interpalpebral lens doesn't work, there are always soft lenses.

- If this isn't a lid effect, the sag of the lens should be increased by increasing the BOZD (and probably the TD) or steepening the BOZR. Either has the effect of making the fit steeper.

- If the fluorescein pattern indicates an aligned lens but the lens moves too much in a vertical plane a lens with a bigger BOZD may be more stable, but you should flatten the BOZR to maintain alignment. In general, an increase in BOZD of 0.5 mm will require a flattening of the BOZR of 0.05 mm to create a "clinically equivalent fit." Remember that initial lacrimation will exaggerate movement, so allow the lens to settle before changing anything.

- A high-riding lens can be modified to reduce lid influence by one or more of the following methods:

  1. **Reduce total diameter**.
  2. **Truncate the lens**. In other words chop a bit off. Most high-riding lenses have minus power, so truncation tends to remove a portion of the thickest part of the lens. This will generally rotate to the top owing to the way the upper lid squeezes the lens, which has the evocative title of the "melon seed effect."
  3. **Lenticulation** of the lens will thin the edge of a minus lens. It is applied to most lenses these days as a standard characteristic, but it might be worth checking.
  4. **Prism ballast** can be added, either alone or with lenticulation. It is also possible to weight the lens with a platinum insert.
  5. A material with greater specific gravity, or a lens of the same material made with greater center thickness, will tend to drop more. It will also flex less, which is a good thing. However, it will transmit less oxygen, which is less good.

- A lens that drops can be more difficult to improve, but try the following:
  1. A larger TD will give the upper lid more lens to grab. However, it will also make the lens heavier unless the design is modified.
  2. Lenticulation. Most dropping lenses have plus power. Lenticulation will reduce the overall weight and move the center of gravity back a bit. Both may help, and the center thickness will be reduced, thus boosting the oxygen transmission.
  3. Use a negative or parallel surface carrier, which thickens up the edge and gives the lid more to grab.
  4. A lens made of a material of lower specific gravity may hold up better.
  5. Check the periphery, as it may be grounding on the upper areas of the cornea.

Troubleshooting astigmatic fits will be considered in the next chapter.

Reference

Van der Worp E, de Brabander J (2005) Contact lens fitting today. Part 1 Modern RGP lens fitting. *Optometry Today* July 15: 27–32.

5
RGP lenses for astigmatism

Introduction

There are two reasons why toric RGP lenses are used. The more common of these is to allow a satisfactory physical fit of the lens on an astigmatic cornea in cases where a spherical lens will not center well or results in too much edge standoff in one meridian. Secondly, we may need to correct residual or induced astigmatism in order for the patient to achieve a satisfactory standard of vision.

About a third of the population has ocular astigmatism over 0.75D and some 7% have an astigmatic element over 2.00D. However, about half of the population have a significantly astigmatic cornea and in over half of these the astigmatism is not symmetrically distributed over the cornea.

Improvements in the design of soft toric lenses and the emergence of toric silicone hydrogel lenses have impacted on the fitting of RGP lenses generally, and soft toric lenses tend to be the first choice these days when correcting astigmatism, especially if the cylinder axis is against the rule or oblique. However, there are still times when a toric RGP lens should be considered. Irregular astigmatism or unusual topography produced by keratoconus or other anomalies of the cornea may have a better visual outcome when RGPs are used, owing to the ability of the tear film to correct irregularities and the greater facility for customization of the lens parameters.

Because of their comparative rarity in all but specialized practices, practitioners tend to approach RGP torics with a degree of trepidation, but there are some mitigating factors to consider. Some candidates for RGP torics are existing RGP wearers who are already adapted to rigid lens wear. They may have spherical PMMA or similar lenses on an astigmatic cornea, but when more oxygen-permeable (and flexible) lenses are fitted, increased lens flexure requires that a toric lens be used to give a satisfactory visual result. When fitting RGP torics to a patient who has not previously worn contact lenses, remember the patient is likely to be well motivated as the alternatives will not correct their vision sufficiently well. Therefore, practitioners should not be afraid of these lenses, although patient expectations should be managed. Toric lenses may need more appointments to achieve an optimal result as factors such as lid influence can be difficult to predict. If the patient is prepared for this from the outset any loss of confidence which might occur if it takes some time to adjust the axis will be avoided. Once in a while, you may get lucky with the first lens that you try, and you can then bask in the acclaim that your outstanding clinical skill will deserve.

Fitting an astigmatic cornea with spherical lenses

The simplest method of fitting an astigmatic cornea, and therefore the one usually tried first, is to use a lens with a spherical or non-toroidal aspherical back surface. Generally, a corneal cylinder up to 3.00D (but 1.50D is probably realistic) may be worth a try with spherical lenses. Sometimes this works very well, but when it doesn't one or more of the following problems will have arisen:

1. The lens will not center properly. In cases of "with the rule" astigmatism the lens may rock back and forth along the steeper corneal meridian or simply drop. With "against the rule" or oblique axes the lens may go sideways. Soft torics may be the best lenses in these cases.
2. The edge clearance along the steeper corneal meridian is excessive. This can be uncomfortable, and interaction between the lens and lid edges can decenter the lens. With corneas showing against the rule astigmatism the horizontal meridian may have excessive edge clearance, leading to 3 and 9 o'clock staining and eventual formation of dellen. Bubble formation under the edge of the lens is common and may cause dimple veiling or annoying visual effects.
3. Historically, PMMA lenses were fairly resistant to lens flexure, but modern lenses are made thin to maximize oxygen transmission and the materials are inherently more flexible. As a result, they tend to flex more on the eye in response to lid

pressure during the blink cycle. The elastic response of the material will not return the lens to its original shape between blinks, so the lens will tend to conform partially to the underlying corneal toricity. Lens flexure may approach a third of the corneal astigmatism, so once we get beyond a 2.00D corneal cylinder it may cause significant blurring of vision. Flexure may be reduced by either increasing the center thickness of the lens or using a less flexible material. Unfortunately, either method will usually reduce oxygen transmission, as flexibility generally increases with the Dk of the material. When refitting PMMA wearers with more permeable materials, toric lenses may be needed to give a satisfactory visual result.

A number of strategies are used by practitioners to overcome these problems, some more successful than others.

To make the lens center better similar strategies are employed to those used in spherical lens fitting. Manipulation of the lid attachment can be achieved through varying the total diameter, and a steeper lens may center better. **Aspheric** designs are reputed to center better than spherical ones on astigmatic corneas, but we are dealing with a two-edged sword here. If they do center on the visual axis the visual result is likely to be excellent, but if they fail to do this they will induce astigmatism in the tear layer and the vision is likely to be both poor and variable.

To reduce excessive edge clearance consider the following:

1. Selecting a smaller BOZD. The smaller the diameters, the smaller the difference in sags between the primary meridians. Lenses with TDs of 9.00 or less may be used, but they may be uncomfortable or unstable as a result of interaction between the lens edge and the lid margins.
2. Steepening the BOZR. Various formulae are in use, and all involve choosing a BOZR which is some way (typically a third or half-way) between the principal meridians rather than fitting on flattest K. The idea is to reduce the edge clear-ance. The problem is that it doesn't actually work. If the flatter corneal meridian is fitted too steep, the effect is to push the

whole lens away from the eye as the primary sag along this meridian is increased. The result is that the edge clearance will still be excessive in the steeper corneal meridian, but we will now have central pooling as well. Steepening may improve the centration of the lens, though not always.

3. The **toric periphery**. Provided the lens is centering well the BOZR can be left unchanged while the peripheral curves are ordered in toric form. The peripheral curves ordered for each principal meridian correspond to those that we would order if we were fitting a lens to a spherical cornea of the same radius. For example, suppose we were fitting an astigmatic cornea with the following Ks:

$$8.00 @ 180$$
$$7.60 @ 90$$

If we choose a BOZR of 8.00 and a TD of 9.20

For the flatter meridian we might order:
8.00:7.00 / 8.80:7.80 / 9.90:8.60 / 11.00:9.20

For the steeper meridian it might be:
7.60:7.00 / 8.30:7.80 / 9.20:8.60 / 10.00:9.20

The toric periphery lens would be ordered as:
8.00:7.00 / 8.80 × 8.30:7.80 / 9.90 × 9.20:8.60 / 11.00 × 10.00:9.20

Should the lens fail to center well, rather more drastic action is required, and the usual remedy would be to use a full **back surface toric.**

Back surface torics

The simplest approach to this is to get the manufacturer to do the donkey work. In general they require accurate refraction results and keratometry readings to two decimal places and back vertex distance (e.g. 7.63 mm @ 125, 8.02 @ 35). From this information, most manufacturers can use computer programs that take into account the refractive index of the lens material to produce a lens that will usually work first time.

The other way to do it would be to extend the process outlined above for a toric periphery, effectively fitting each principal meridian as if it were a spherical cornea of the same radius. For the example above this would result in the following back surface:

8.00 × 7.60:7.00 / 8.80 × 8.30:7.80 / 9.90 × 9.20:8.60 / 11.00 × 10.00:9.20

The resulting lens should center and show a similar fluorescein pattern to a spherical lens on a spherical cornea (Figure 5.1).

However, while the tear lens behind a spherical lens on an astigmatic cornea will effectively correct the corneal astigmatism, once we use a back surface toric the optics become more complicated.

Let's consider a cornea with Ks of 8.00 along 180 and 7.60 along 90.

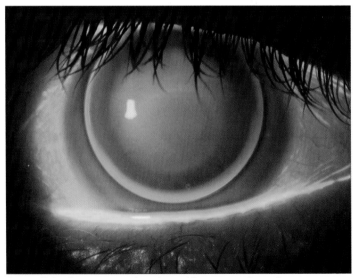

Figure 5.1 Appearance of a spherical lens on a spherical cornea

The rule of thumb is that each 0.1 mm difference in radius corresponds to 0.5D of corneal astigmatism, though a simpler way to measure it on a patient is to use the dioptric scale on the keratometer. Either way, we have 2.00D of corneal astigmatism here with an axis of 180°. Were we to fit a spherical BOZR here this astigmatism would be effectively fully corrected, as the refractive indices of the tear film and cornea are very similar. However, if we fit a back surface toric the refractive index of the lens material will be significantly higher, and the result will be that the corneal astigmatism will be over-corrected.

The **induced astigmatism** that the back surface of the lens will create can be calculated by the following formula:

$$I = \frac{n - n'}{r_1} - \frac{n - n'}{r_2}$$

where
I = induced astigmatism
n = refractive index of tears (1.336)
n' = refractive index of contact lens material (1.480, for example)
r_1 = steeper radius of curvature in meters (0.0076 here)
r_2 = flatter radius of curvature in meters (0.0080 in this case).

$$I = \frac{1.336 - 1.480}{0.0076} - \frac{1.336 - 1.480}{0.0080} = 0.95D$$

If the patient's ocular astigmatism is equal to their corneal astigmatism, we have a problem, because the **residual astigmatism** (ocular astigmatism minus corneal astigmatism) will be zero. As the induced astigmatism is nearly a diopter, we will be over-correcting the astigmatism by the same amount.

The **1-2-3 rule** gives an approximation of the effect of using a back surface toric. If we work the equivalent of a 2.00D corneal cylinder (i.e. about 0.4 mm difference in radii between principal meridians) onto the back surface of a PMMA lens it will modify the residual astigmatism found by over-refraction over a spherical lens by 1.00D. When measured on a focimeter, a 3.00D cylinder will be measured. This is due to the differences in the refractive indices of the lens material and air and those of the cornea and tear film. For RGP materials of lower refractive index than PMMA the values are slightly reduced.

Where the use of a back surface toric induces an inappropriate correction there are two strategies to consider:

1. **Selecting back surface radii for their optical effect**. If we reduce the difference between the two principal meridians of the lens, the induced astigmatism will be reduced, but to reduce it to zero we are back to a spherical back surface. However, in practice, there is usually some residual astigmatism to correct and by slightly flattening the steeper meridian a satisfactory optical outcome can be achieved in many cases, provided the ocular astigmatism exceeds corneal astigmatism. (If it is the other way round, see below.) Tear exchange may also be enhanced if the steeper lens meridian is flattened slightly, especially if it is the vertical one. This was a common practice when PMMA lenses were in use, but it can result in increased lens flexure when using the more flexible modern materials.

2. **Toroidal front surface** (bitoric).

Bitoric lenses

The simplest form of bitoric lens is the **"compensated"** or **"spherical power equivalent"** type. These are designed for the situation where corneal and ocular astigmatism correspond. The front surface toricity exists purely to eliminate the induced astigmatism that the back surface creates. When placed upon the eye the over-refraction will be spherical. The lens can also rotate on the eye without causing blurring of vision as the toricity of the tear lens will compensate for rotation of the front surface cylinder. To prescribe these, it is necessary to work out the induced astigmatism and order a counteracting cylinder for the front surface. However, the lab will probably be able to work this out on computer for you. If not, there are computer programs available from a number of sources.

"Alignment" bitorics have a front surface that corrects both induced and residual astigmatism. The correction for residual astigmatism will be "aligned" along one of the principal meridians of the lens. Because there is a correction for residual astigmatism these lenses cannot be allowed to rotate excessively, or the vision will be affected.

"Oblique" bitorics may be used where the axes of the corneal and ocular astigmatism do not correspond. The axes of the front surface need to be set differently to the principal meridians of the back surface. These rather complex lenses are only rarely needed, particularly since the emergence of successful soft and silicone hydrogel torics. They also need to be stabilized against rotation.

Rotation and stabilization

Once we have a front surface cylinder, some means has to be found to stabilize its axis, or the vision will be rather variable. During the blink cycle closure of the lids proceeds from outer to inner canthus ("the zipper effect"). The upper lid moves vertically down to close the eye, then up again to open it. The lower lid, however, does not move vertically, so as it tightens it imparts a force on the lens that will tend to spin the lower part of the lens nasally.

To counteract this effect a number of strategies may be employed:

1. A back surface toric fitted in alignment with a toroidal cornea will resist spin. The more toricity the better the effect, so it is easier to fit patients with higher corneal and lower ocular astigmatism than it is to fit those whose ocular astigmatism is higher.
2. Prism ballast may be incorporated, typically 1–2 Δ. The base of the prism will align itself at the lowest point of the lens as a result of the "melon seed principle," whereby the squeeze pressure of the upper lid expels the thinnest part of the lens (the prism apex) last. The disadvantage of prism ballast is that the lower edge is thicker so the lens may be less comfortable. The lens will also be heavier, which can cause it to drop.

3. Platinum weights can be inserted into the lens. These will align themselves at the lowest point of the lens owing to gravity, but they may also cause the lens to drop, but get real.

4. Truncation of the lower, and sometimes upper, part of the lens may allow the lid margins to impart desirable spin on the lens, especially if combined with prism ballast. However, the edge may cause unacceptable discomfort.

Troubleshooting

Patient dissatisfaction with RGP torics will usually be on the grounds of poor vision or discomfort.

Poor vision

Vision may not meet expectations if the spectacle Rx or keratometer readings are inaccurate. The former can be a problem if the practitioner fitting the lenses did not do the last spectacle refraction, and when fitting torics it is always a good idea to verify the spectacle Rx for yourself. The K readings should also be checked carefully, particularly the orientation of the principal corneal meridians to ensure that they match the axis of the ocular correction. If they do not, an oblique bitoric lens may be required, or a soft toric lens.

On a lens with back surface astigmatism, the principal meridians of the back surface should align themselves with those of the cornea, but lid influence may modify this, especially if the corneal astigmatism is low. It may be possible to change the orientation of any prism ballast used, or fine-tune the shape and orientation of a truncation to improve this, but we are entering the domain of the specialist practitioner here and the process may be a prolonged and expensive one. Soft torics present an attractive option here.

The axis may be inclined to spin during the blink cycle, and some patients tolerate this better than others. Manipulation of prism ballast or lens shape may work, but again soft torics start to look like the best option.

Discomfort

Patients new to RGPs will have to adapt to the sensation that the edge of the lens imparts to the lids, and even established rigid lens wearers may struggle, given that toric lenses generally have thicker edges, especially if prism-ballasted and truncated. Some patients will simply never adapt to this and a soft toric option may be the answer.

6
RGP contact lenses in presbyopia

Introduction

In the good old days, when bread tasted like bread and contact lenses were rigid, it used to be quite possible for the busy practitioner to pretend that multifocal contact lenses didn't exist, or at least could be regarded as the exclusive preserve of the contact lens nerd. A few specialized practitioners did much of the little multifocal fitting that was attempted. Those collecting case records for specialist qualifications usually did the rest. Many swore never to repeat the experience given any choice in the matter, as the process at the time was both time-consuming and had a success rate that could be politely termed modest.

This state of affairs couldn't last forever and multifocals are now an area that any practitioner involved in the prescribing and fitting of contact lenses must address. In the UK, we are told, as in all developed countries, the population is aging. People have always aged, as the alternative is much worse, but now people tend to continue to do so for rather longer. There is a growing percentage of the population aged over 45 years, and this trend is continuing. In 1991, 37.1% of the UK population was over 45 years old, and it is projected that by 2011 this figure will have risen to 43.5%. The average age of the population has increased from 34.1 years in 1971 to 38.2 years in 2002, and is expected to rise to 43.3 years by 2031. The trend is a result of both a reduction in birth rate and a population with greater life expectancy. The number of people requiring optical correction of their presbyopia is also therefore increasing. Realistically, not all of this age group will be interested in contact lenses. The very elderly may consider contact lenses to be new-fangled things – like computers or portable telephones – and refuse to have anything to do with them. Realistically the 45–65 group is probably the target market for multifocal contact lenses, and most of the first-time multifocals will be at the lower end of the age range. They will include both current contact lens wearers and those who are purely spectacle wearers, although the latter group will contain some individuals who have worn lenses in the past. The onset of presbyopia used to be one of those events that precipitated drop-out from contact lens wear because of the previous lack of a viable multifocal option, and there are some previous wearers who would like to give contact lenses another go. This group, and the group of current contact lens wearers negotiating the onset of presbyopia at the moment, will contain an unusually high proportion of RGP wearers compared to the normal run of contact lens patients seen in practice. We used to fit more RGPs than we do now, and approximately 40% of all RGP wearers are over 45 years of age. RGP lenses tend to correct astigmatism rather more easily than soft multifocals do and often give better near vision as a result, so they may also be useful for previous soft lens wearers. Those patients who approach multifocal lenses without prior contact lens experience are often making the same sort of "lifestyle" purchase that brings Harley-Davidsons to middle-aged executives. The early presbyope often has more disposable income than at any period before or since. The kids have been packed off to higher education or gainful employment, the mortgage has been paid off, and their career is peaking. A little pampering is required, and multifocal contact lenses can be a key ingredient in the attempt to regain lost youth, or at least its illusion.

In many ways it is fortunate that it is the early presbyope who usually wants contact lenses. As any practitioner will have been told far too many times, "old age doesn't come alone." Changes in the tear film, conjunctival folds, and slackening of the eyelids can all complicate contact lens fitting, and the presbyopic patient is far more likely to be on long-term medication, much of which (e.g. β-blockers and hormone replacement therapy) can contribute to dry eye. On the other hand, some of the long-term contact lens wearers may bear the evidence of their misspent youth, which may influence the choice of multifocal by the practitioner.

Presbyopia

Presbyopia is an age-related progressive loss of accommodative amplitude. In 1909, Helmholtz described accommodation as occurring when contraction of the ciliary muscle releases tension in the zonular fibers. In the young eye, the elasticity of the lens and capsule allows the lens to become more spherical, and the increased curvature of the surfaces provides extra positive power. When the ciliary muscle relaxes, the elasticity of the zonular fibers and the choroid pull it back into its resting state, This reintroduces tension on the zonular fibers at the edge of the lens, causing the lens to flatten. This model, though challenged, has largely been confirmed by imaging techniques. There have been two main schools of thought on the cause of presbyopia. Lenticular theories concentrate on age-related changes to the lens substance, capsule and zonular fibers. Extralenticular theories consider changes to the ciliary muscle, connective tissue and choroid. A multifactorial approach is now becoming popular, incorporating both lenticular and extralenticular elements. To a certain extent, the precise mechanism is not as important to the contact lens practitioner as it is to those involved in the evolution of presbyopic refractive surgery.

The onset of the processes that produce presbyopia is thought to be early in life, probably soon after the eye stops growing. Its culmination occurs around the age of 55 years when no actual accommodation is occurring. But the age at which any individual has to bow to the inevitable depends on some other factors. Patients with small pupils have a greater depth of focus, so they may be able to focus closer at a greater age, at least in a good light. The resting pupil diameter does tend to reduce with age, but considerable variation may be produced by pathology and medication as well as ambient light conditions. Another major factor in the age of onset is height. Tall people have longer arms, and habitually hold reading material at a greater working distance. The demands of near vision vary greatly between individuals and the patient who primarily works at a VDU and rarely reads may not be troubled for some years after a colleague who reads novels. Even the font size of the chosen daily paper may influence that moment when we all realize that presbyopia doesn't just happen to other people.

Myopes with medium to high spectacle prescriptions are often rather smug when their hyperopic and emmetropic friends submit to presbyopia. They can delay the inevitable by exploiting the power change induced by looking obliquely through the lower part of the lens. In effect they have a free reading addition long before they have to admit to needing one, and the diopter or so provided by this can be further enhanced by pulling the spectacles down the nose. This increases the BVD and thus decreases the effective negative power of the spectacles. However, if such a patient decides to go for contact lenses they can receive an unpleasant shock when they attempt to read, since neither of these strategies will be available. To add to their woes, accommodative demand is greater with contact lenses than it is with a myopic spectacle correction. This should of course result in a greater amount of accommodative convergence becoming available to reduce their exophoria. This is just as well, as convergence demand is also increased, and the rather useful base-in prism that their spectacles used to provide has disappeared. To summarize, if we fit a myopic early presbyope with contact lenses we may induce near vision problems associated with both feeble accommodation and/or decompensated exophoria. The situation may be different if the myope habitually reads or uses a VDU without spectacles. In this case correcting the myopia with contact lenses could place considerable extra demands on accommodation, and this in turn could precipitate an esophoria. Given that the negative fusional reserves appear to reduce with age, decompensation is a possibility here. In comparison, hyperopes can usually switch to contact lenses relatively easily, though they can miss the extra magnification that spectacles provide and this may be reflected in their visual acuity. They will gain in terms of visual field size, however.

When a reading addition is introduced, the accommodative demand for a given distance will be reduced, and with it the amount of accommodative convergence available. Therefore the fusional reserves must be adequate to ensure comfortable binocular vision. The incorporation of horizontal prism in a multifocal contact lens is not a viable option.

RGP contact lenses in presbyopia

For the presbyopic RGP wearer who wishes to continue with lenses there are a number of options:

1. **Single vision contact lenses** for distance and the use of spectacles for near vision as required. This does rather defeat the original object of contact lens wear, but it is nevertheless a popular option with both practitioner and patient. It is simple, and the visual acuity obtained is usually excellent. It is also cost-effective, as many patients use ready-made spectacles to supplement their distance contact lenses. However, the binocular considerations outlined above may cause difficulties if the lenses are not properly centered for the patient.

2. **Monovision** describes the process of fitting lenses to correct one eye for distance and one eye for near. Studies have shown that this method enjoys higher success rates than multifocal contact lens fitting, but it doesn't suit everyone.

3. **Multifocal contact lenses** can be divided into two main categories: alternating vision and simultaneous vision. A number of subdivisions exist within each category, each with some advantages and disadvantages and each allows certain parameters to be varied to optimize the effect for the individual patient. That said, it is one of life's little ironies that those who are best able to work with the variations are the very people who need them least. The over-riding requirement in a potential multifocal wearer is flexibility, as all of them are likely to result in some visual compromise at distance or near, or both. The patient who can adapt to this is usually relatively easy to fit, though it is probably the same patient who could cheerfully adapt to progressive spectacle lenses, reading glasses or any of the other types of presbyopic correction. On the other hand, the detail-obsessed and inflexible patient should be avoided, and there is anecdotal evidence that such people tend to have a high probability of an inadequate tear film, especially those who turn up with a list. If a patient cannot adapt to the first type of lens chosen it might be bad luck. When they can't quite get on with the second or third lens it is more likely to be a psychological trait and it is a wise practitioner who can quit when they are behind.

Alternating vision lenses are required to *translate*, or move relative to the pupil. These are almost invariably RGP lenses, as on

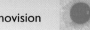

the whole it is relatively easy to get an RGP to decenter. The advantage to this approach is that all of the light entering the pupil area is focused for the same distance, so the vision should suffer less degradation. The downside is the skill and time required to fit them well. Alternating lenses are generally fitted using the lid-attachment model.

Lenses in the **simultaneous vision** category are expected to stay pretty much where they are, and soft lens multifocal designs are of this type. They are normally easier to fit but involve more visual compromise as a significant proportion of the light entering the pupil from the object of regard will not focus in the retinal plane. The simplest form of simultaneous lens has concentric zones of distance and near power, but most modern lenses have aspheric surfaces, allowing a progressive power function analogous to a varifocal spectacle lens. There is some debate as to how some of these RGP multifocals work. It has been customary to classify aspheric multifocals in the simultaneous category, and there will be some element of this, but all of them need some translation to work properly. Aspheric lenses seem to work by a combination of alternating and simultaneous vision, with the exact blend varying from patient to patient. On the other hand, so do progressive spectacle lenses.

Monovision

The basic principle in monovision is to correct one eye for distance and one for near, and on the whole it works quite well. Estimates of the success rate vary between 50% and 86% depending on the criteria used to define success, but numerous studies have consistently found monovision to be rather more successful than multifocal fitting, and it is generally a simpler process. Furthermore, conventional single vision lenses can be used, and these will usually fit better and involve less physiological compromise than any multifocal.

The ability to suppress detrimental blur information is significantly higher in successful monovision patients, but predicting who has this ability in a clinical setting is challenging.

For a thorough review of the literature see Evans (2006). Alternating squinters are ideal, as they are well practiced in suppression of the non-fixating eye. Strong ocular dominance may be an asset when the dominant eye is fully corrected but could be a distraction when the other eye is the one being used. Patients who report a high level of "ghosting" during a monovision contact lens trial may be poor candidates for monovision. Other characteristics that might indicate a more guarded prognosis include age and psychological traits. Older patients tend to be less successful as they may be less adaptable and they also need higher reading additions to see clearly. Structured, detail-oriented and pessimistic people are less successful than holistic, adaptable optimistic ones. In other words, beware the list-maker.

Which eye to correct for distance is also a challenging question. Conventionally, the distance correction is applied to the "dominant" eye determined by a sighting test, but this does not guarantee the best visual result. Alternatively, the +2.00 test described by Michaud et al (1995) may be employed. Essentially this consists of placing a +2.00 lens in front of each eye in turn, and comparing the distance vision. If the vision is best with the +2.00 before the left eye, then the right eye is considered the dominant eye for distance. This is fairly reliable if distance vision is a priority, but this is not always the case. The best way to establish whether monovision will work and which way round to correct the eyes is to try it. This is best done in the form of an extended trial over several days, so that the patient may experience the effect at home and in the workplace. Disposable soft lenses make this a relatively inexpensive process.

Those patients who do not adapt to monovision may encounter a number of problems. Blur may be experienced by those who do not suppress it efficiently, especially at night where glare or haloes can make night driving difficult. About a third of monovision patients report this. Stereopsis will be adversely affected, yet this rarely seems to be noticed by patients. However, it may be worth mentioning to them as a precaution against future litigation. Finally, decompensation of binocular vision is a rare complication, probably because most of those patients likely to be affected have some ability to suppress.

Partial monovision

Full correction of the near vision may be impractical. Pardhan and Gilchrist (1990) found that at a point between 1.00 and 1.50D the eyes crossed over from binocular summation to binocular inhibition. When binocular summation is occurring, the binocular contrast sensitivity is about 40% higher than the monocular. With binocular inhibition the binocular sensitivity is lower than the monocular. This correlates well with anecdotal evidence from contact lens practitioners and refractive surgeons that adds below +1.50 work better. However, a high add might help to stabilize blur suppression in some cases, so there may be exceptions to the rule.

Enhanced monovision

A variation on the monovision theme is to fit one eye with a single vision lens and the other with a multifocal. Usually this involves a single vision distance lens in the dominant eye and a multifocal in the other. The idea is to improve distance vision, usually for driving, while allowing at least casual near vision. This may be a useful option for the early presbyope, going over to bilateral bifocal correction later on. Other variations include a SV near/distance-biased multifocal combination and a slightly over-plussed SV distance/intermediate-biased multifocal for a VDU user.

Modified monovision

This involves fitting both eyes with a multifocal lens, but biasing one eye more for distance and one eye for near. This can be achieved by adjusting the power of the lens. Under-correcting the reading addition will bias a lens towards distance vision, and over-plussing the distance correction puts the bias towards near vision. Alternatively a different design of multifocal may be used in each eye. A distance center lens in one eye and a near center lens in the other is a popular combination.

Choosing a rigid bifocal lens

The current Association of Contact Lens Manufacturers (ACLM) manual lists over 30 different options in multifocal RGP lenses, so where do we start? We need to consider both the physical characteristics of the patient and their lifestyle, but it is important to manage patient expectations from the outset. Multifocal fitting may be relatively prolonged and therefore potentially expensive in terms of both chair time and lenses and the patient should not expect a quick fix. It is fortunate that most potential candidates for these lenses are existing RGP wearers who will be well adapted to rigid lens wear, as lenses on an unadapted patient rarely behave on the eye in the same way as they will eventually.

Provided that they translate successfully, alternating designs will generally give the best acuity at near because all of the available light is being focused at the same point. Simultaneous designs split the light between more than one focal point, so contrast sensitivity is compromised at all distances and for prolonged reading supplementary spectacles may be needed. However, certain patients will present a challenge when fitting alternating bifocals:

1. Lower lids that are positioned below the limbus may compromise lens translation. Patients with this configuration are best fitted with an aspheric design.
2. Against the rule and oblique astigmatism may cause the lens to translate sideways or eccentrically. Soft multifocals may be an easier route to take. With the rule astigmatism can often be helpful to translating multifocals.
3. Patients who undertake extensive arm's length visual tasks may be better off with aspheric designs, as they offer both a progressive focus and some simultaneous vision rather than the fixed distance and near of a purely alternating design.

Given the typical profile of a new RGP multifocal fitting, there is a high probability that the patient will spend regular time on a computer, and anyone who cooks will find intermediate vision an essential. However, there are trifocal variants on most bifocal designs.

4. Patients who need to see at near in a variety of positions of gaze will also do better with a simultaneous design. Mechanics, electricians, plumbers and librarians are obvious examples. On the other hand this function may not be useful to all. A weekend cricketer fielding in the deep might not appreciate it at all when trying to catch a "skyer."

5. Patients who are particularly sensitive to lid sensation will struggle with translating lenses.

"Simultaneous" designs are generally easier to fit than alternating designs, but there are some patients who might be tricky:

1. Large pupils can give rise to poor visual acuity and flare with both aspheric and concentric simultaneous designs. Anything over about 6 mm is unpromising.

2. Decentration of any sort will result in induced astigmatism and reduced vision with an aspheric lens. Some patients will show a corneal apex that is superior to the pupil center. A translating design will work better here.

3. Patients who are picky about the quality of vision may be unhappy with any simultaneous design, particularly in low light conditions. However, they will possibly have issues with any form of multifocal lens.

Alternating vision bifocals

This type of lens is usually only available in RGP form, though attempts have been made to develop a soft version. The lens is fitted so that in primary gaze the patient is looking through the distance portion. When the patient looks down to read, the lens is held up on the lower lid, which does not move down at the same rate as the eye.

The lens usually will incorporate prism ballast and truncation to assist segment positioning. However, photographic evidence suggests that the lower lid accounts for only about 1 mm of the translation. Upper lid attachment accounts for the rest. In downgaze, the patient will be looking through the near vision portion of the lens, provided the lens translates perfectly. However, in real life things are rarely quite perfect, and it is common for at least one of a patient's lenses to translate only partially. With a fully translating lens the vision obtained should be excellent, but partial translation may compromise this slightly. Solid designs are cut from a single piece of material and various segment shapes are possible. However, unless the distance and near optical centers are made to coincide (monocentric design), image jump will occur when the patient changes between distance and near vision. Monocentric lenses have a straight division between the distance and near portion, and look rather like a miniature executive bifocal. Probably the most familiar example would be the Tangent Streak (Fused Kontacts, Missouri) design. This lens is available with a range of additions (0.75–4.00D), bifocal heights and prism ballasts (1.75–4.00$^\Delta$).

To fit this lens, a diagnostic fitting set is by far the best way, but with the current concern over the transmission of variant Creutzfeldt–Jakob disease (vCJD), an alternative is to order an initial lens empirically and use it as a diagnostic lens to refine the fitting. The base curves shown in Table 6.1 are recommended.

The BOZR needs to be flatter than the superior cornea, or translation will be inhibited. The lens should center a little low on the cornea with the segment ideally positioned 1.3 mm below the pupil center. On many patients this will mean that the near segment impinges on the pupil during distance gaze, but up to 30% coverage by the near segment may be tolerated without compromising distance vision unacceptably. In downgaze the lens should move up, overlapping the sclera.

The following challenges may present:

1. **Discomfort** is fairly common, as these lenses may be heavy and thick, especially on the lower edge. It may be possible to

Table 6.1 **Recommended base curves for alternating vision bifocals**

Corneal astigmatism	BOZR
0	0.2 mm flatter than K
0.50D (0.1 mm)	0.1 mm flatter than K
1.00D (0.2 mm)	No steeper than K of more than $1/4$ astigmatism

thin the edges somewhat. A thinner, fused-segment bifocal such as the Fluoroperm ST may help, but the alternative would be to consider a simultaneous vision design.

2. **3 and 9 o'clock staining** is also a potential problem with thick lenses, as the lids are held away from the cornea. Changing the diameter and/or thinning the edges may be a solution.

3. **Lateral decentration** may be improved by increasing the TD of the lens and by steepening the BOZR.

4. **Rotation of the segment** will result in poor near vision. This is caused by the fact that the lower lid moves transversely during the blink cycle towards the inner canthus. This will tend to spin the lens so that the near segment will move nasally. A number of strategies may be employed to counteract this:
   (a) Flattening the BOZR may help.
   (b) Changing the prism axis will help if the rotation is stable, but not with an unstable lens. Changes are rarely more than 20°.
   (c) Increasing the prism ballast will steady an unstable lens.
   (d) Decreasing the TD may help, but only if upper lid capture is the cause.
   (e) Changing the orientation or shape of the truncation may work, but here we are at the point where art takes over from science. Modify a bit at a time, and see what happens before making major modifications.

5. **Inadequate translation** may have a number of causes:
   (a) The back surface fit of the lens may be wrong. The lens

may be too big and catching on the upper cornea or sclera during downgaze. The BOZR may be too steep, or the peripheral clearance inadequate. Careful observance of the fluorescein pattern during downgaze, with the upper lid lifted, may reveal the fault. The lens can be translated manually by pushing it up with the lower lid. Checking the fit should always be the first step with a misbehaving lens.

(b) Lid attachment may be inadequate as a result of a slack upper lid or a lens that is too small or has too thin an edge. In this case, increasing the TD or thickening the edge with a negative carrier may be effective.

6. **Poor distance vision** may be caused by interference from a near segment that is too high, or by a high-riding lens.

(a) A high segment can be lowered by increasing the truncation, so when ordering lenses initially it is wise to aim a little high.

(b) A high-riding lens may be lowered by increasing the prism or reducing the TD.

(c) If the lens is held too high by a tight upper lid, the Lifestyle lens may work well.

7. **Slow return** after a blink may cause a delay in distance focus. Increasing the prism or reducing the TD will make the lens recover faster.

Until recently, a popular alternative was the Fluoroperm ST (Paragon Vision Sciences). This had an encapsulated flat-topped segment analogous to a fused D-segment spectacle lens and it was a thinner, lighter lens than the Tangent Streak. However, it appears to be unobtainable at present.

The Presbylite II (Pro Cornea, Netherlands) has a triangular near segment with a small aspheric (and therefore progressive) area at the top. It is monocentric and all of the optical surfaces are cut on the front surface, so a back surface toric is possible. It can be obtained in any power combination, and is usually made in Boston XO, which gives it respectable oxygen permeability. The lens is thin for a multifocal and has no truncation.

Aspheric and concentric designs

These lenses are becoming more popular in recent years as they are more comfortable than purely alternating designs, since they do not need their prism ballast or truncations. Modern CNC (computer numeric controlled) lathes allow complex surface to be manufactured very accurately. All of these lenses need to translate somewhat in order to work well, but they do not rely entirely on translation for their effect.

Back surface aspherics use the tear film to provide the reading addition. The central part of the back surface of the lens is steeper than the cornea and flattens at a predetermined rate towards the periphery. In downgaze the lens translates and this changes the shape of the post-lens tear film, increasing the positive power. The original Quasar Plus (no. 7) lens was a back surface aspheric, but front surface asphericity was added when it became apparent that the addition created by the back surface asphericity alone was insufficient. The precise addition obtained with a back surface aspheric is a little unpredictable, since it will depend on both the patient's corneal topography and the degree to which the lens translates. The former uncertainty has been addressed by computer algorithms that can generate a predictable progressive power for a given cornea from topographical analysis (e.g. Z-Wave). However, to use this system, a topographer and design software are essentials, and a certain amount of patient footfall would be needed to justify the investment.

The lens is fitted to provide mid-peripheral alignment, with the fluorescein pattern showing central clearance. The trick with this lens is to get it to translate enough to provide good near vision without making it unstable. If the lens is moving properly it is rarely necessary to add extra near power, so it is always worth attending to the fit first. Simply adding extra near power may improve near vision, but often at the cost of some blurring at distance. The steep central fit of this type of lens creates potential for corneal molding and consequent spectacle blur. This can be minimized by the use of high Dk materials, but patients who alternate between contact lenses and spectacles may find this challenging.

The Lifestyle (Cantor and Nissel) lens is also fitted with central clearance, the bearing surface being a secondary aspheric curve 1.2 mm wide. The "equivalent base curve" is chosen up to 0.1 mm flatter than flattest K as the usual starting point, and a lens which is too steep will not translate successfully. There are two TDs available: 9.00 and 9.50. The 9.00 is the usual starting point, but if this does not center high enough a larger, flatter lens may help. The reading addition is limited to a nominal +1.75 so it is best suited to early presbyopes, especially computer users. A tightish upper lid is helpful for both adequate translation and stability, and with the rule astigmatism is also a useful characteristic for a prospective patient. Existing RGP wearers whose lenses ride high tend to be successful with this type of lens. However, those with low-riding lenses or large pupils may be less pleased.

Front surface aspheric designs avoid this effect as their back surfaces may be designed purely for physiological effect, like their single vision cousins. Indeed many of these lenses have a back surface geometry based on single vision designs. This makes selection of base curves rather easy, especially if the patient is already wearing the single vision equivalent. It also makes patient adaptation easier, as the multifocal lenses are quite similar in feel to the single vision ones. The Profile Additions lens from Davis Thomas has a front surface incorporating SAM (spherical aberration management) and a back surface based on the polynomial aspheric design used on the Profile single vision lens. This is a **center-distance lens**, as are most RGPs, although it is possible to construct a lens with the greatest plus power in the center (**center-near**). However, given that RGPs tend to translate, a center-near lens, though a popular configuration in soft multifocals, is of limited use.

The Menicon Z lens offers **extended wear capabilities**, and its high oxygen transmission is useful even in conventional daily wear. This is a **concentric multifocal** with three distinct areas worked on the front surface. There is a central distance zone and a peripheral near zone. Between them is an annulus in which the power is progressive from distance to near, giving the lens a progressive capability. In downgaze, the lens is expected to translate about 2 mm. The back surface consists of a large spherical optic zone surrounded by an aspheric periphery, like the single vision version of the lens. The diameter of the distance zone reduces as the reading addition goes up, which is no problem provided the patient does not have unusually large pupils.

References

Evans B (2006) Monovision: a systematic review. *Ophthalmic Physiol. Opt.* (forthcoming)

Michaud L, Tchang JP, Baril C, Gresset J (1995) New perspectives in monovision: a study comparing aspheric with disposable lenses. *Int. Contact Lens Clin.* **22**:203–8.

Pardhan S, Gilchrist J (1990) The effect of monocular defocus on binocular contrast sensitivity. *Ophthalmic Physiol. Opt.* **10**(1):33–6.

7
Keratoconus

Introduction

Keratoconus may be defined as a progressive, non-inflammatory condition which involves thinning of the central cornea and protrusion and distortion of the cornea into a conical shape. The optometrist in general practice may become involved in the diagnosis, fitting and aftercare of keratoconic patients, although most of the care of the more advanced stages is likely to be hospital based. Keratoconus is one of the more challenging areas of contact lens practice and there is something of a gray area about most aspects of the disease, but contact lenses form an important part of the management of this condition.

There is no universally accepted definition of keratoconus and this is reflected in the various estimates of its prevalence within the population, which range from 4 to 230 in every 100 000. Corneal topography has revealed that some patients appear to have a subclinical form of the condition which Amsler termed "keratoconus fruste." This progresses only very slowly and may never seriously inconvenience the patient. Occasionally it may be seen in one eye while the other eye shows more marked abnormality.

The exact etiology is also obscure. It is a little more common in men, particularly those of Asian origin. There is certainly an association with connective tissue disorders and with various syndromes (Crouzon, Ehlers-Danlos, Reiger, Marfan, Leber and Down syndromes to name but a few). There may be an hereditary factor, but most cases appear random. About half of all keratoconics appear to be atopic and this has led to speculation that when these patients rub their eyes to relieve itching they may initiate or exacerbate the disease process through a process of chronic keratocyte apoptosis (programmed cell death). There is evidence that the genetic abnormality for keratoconus occurs on the same gene as those for asthma and eczema.

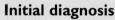

Initial diagnosis

Keratoconus is often diagnosed in young adults who present for routine refraction and typically the first sign detected is an increase in astigmatism, and usually myopia, in one or both eyes. The condition is bilateral but usually asymmetric. At this stage the cornea may appear normal unless corneal topography is investigated, and spectacle correction will give satisfactory vision. Eventually, the astigmatism will show an unfeasibly large increase in degree or axis shift and it may be impossible to obtain a visual acuity that satisfies practitioner or patient.

At this stage a number of other findings may confirm the diagnosis:

1. **Keratometry** will give steep readings and the mires may be distorted.
2. **Retinoscopy** may show a "scissors" reflex.
3. The slit-lamp may reveal the following anomalies:
   (a) **Vogt's striae**: fine white lines in the deep stroma. They are usually vertical but may be oblique. They are stress lines caused by stretching of the corneal lamellae, and if pressure is applied externally to the globe they will disappear.
   (b) Corneal nerves may appear more prominent.

Later signs include the following:

1. **Fleischer's ring** is a brown or green line encircling the base of the cone, though rarely completely. It is formed from an iron-based pigment in the basal epithelium in about 50% of keratoconic patients. It is more easily seen with cobalt blue light.
2. **Corneal thinning** in the central or paracentral areas will be apparent with high magnification and a thin corneal section. Pachymetry may be helpful if available.

3. **Munson's sign** is a bulging of the lower lid when the patient looks down.

4. **Central and paracentral scarring** occur in severe cases, and may be exacerbated by heavy apical touch from RGP lenses.

5. **Ruptures in Descemet's membrane** allow aqueous fluid to leak into the corneal stroma, resulting in **acute hydrops.** The visual acuity drops suddenly and the patient may experience discomfort and excessive lacrimation. The membrane usually repairs within 10 weeks but scarring may ensue. Short-term relief may be provided with hypertonic saline and either patching or a soft bandage contact lens. Severe cases may require penetrating keratoplasty (Figure 7.1).

Early keratoconic changes usually appear as a small area of irregular curvature in the inferior paracentral cornea, but as the

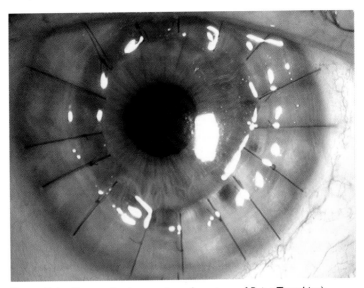

Figure 7.1 Penetrating keratoplasty (courtesy of Brian Tompkins)

condition progresses it may be differentiated into three categories, although a few corneas defy categorization:

1. The **nipple** form has a small central or paracentral ectasia, up to 5 mm in diameter, surrounded by normal cornea. There is sometimes a smaller elevated nodule at the apex. This nodule is rich in fibroblasts and if abraded by lens with heavy apical touch, could result in scarring.
2. The **oval** form is the most common, in which the corneal apex is displaced inferiorly. This inferior steepening may be associated with a corresponding area above the midline which has normal or even flatter than normal curvature. Some contact lens types feature offset peripheral curves that are designed to provide more clearance over the superior cornea. Oval cones tend to have more breaks in Bowman's membrane, more superior pannus formation and more ruptures of Descemet's membrane than nipple cones.
3. The **globus** form involves up to three-quarters of the corneal surface and the mid-peripheral area of normal cornea that surrounds the cone in the other forms is absent.

The best way to find out which form we are dealing with, and indeed to confirm the initial diagnosis, is topographical mapping. If this is not available in-house it is worth seeking elsewhere before attempting fitting contact lenses as it may save a lot of time in the long run. Hospitals often provide such data if they send patients out for fitting in general practice, and most places will have a topographer available locally. In the absence of topographical data the severity of the condition may be indicated by keratometry, and some idea of the type of cone present may be indicated by the use of a Placido disk or similar device:

1. **Mild** keratoconus will have a corneal curvature that will read up to 48D on the power scale.
2. **Moderate** stages will read between 48 and 54D.
3. **Severe** stages will read over 54D.

Management of keratoconus

The management of keratoconus depends on its severity:

1. **Spectacle correction** may give a surprisingly good level of vision in early cases, and the wise practitioner is not in too much of a hurry to get the patient into contact lenses. Keratoconic fitting is tricky for a number of reasons and those patients who obtain a marked improvement in vision with contact lenses are likely to be better motivated to cope with what can be a prolonged and frustrating fitting process.

2. **Soft toric lenses** are rarely fitted, but in early cases may provide adequate vision. Both this option and spectacle correction avoid the increased risk of corneal scarring that RGP lenses may bring.

3. **RGP lenses** are the most common management strategy for more advance keratoconus. The tear film behind a rigid lens is capable of correcting some 90% of corneal astigmatism, be it regular or irregular.

4. **Scleral lenses** used to be the first choice for keratoconus but are now generally only used when RGP lenses cannot provide adequate correction.

5. **"Piggyback" lenses** consist of a rigid lens fitted on top of a soft carrier lens. They may be useful on very irregular corneas where conventional lenses fail to center, but the increased combined lens thickness does not help oxygen transmission.

6. **Hybrid lenses** such as the Softperm (CIBA) consist of an RGP center surrounded by a soft lens skirt, which can aid centration in some cases.

7. **Corneal surgery** may be required by 10–20% of patients eventually.

   (a) **Epikeratoplasty** is a process whereby a lenticule of donor tissue is added to the cornea. The objective is to thicken and flatten the central cornea and reduce astigmatism. This procedure is used on those patients who

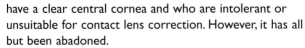
have a clear central cornea and who are intolerant or unsuitable for contact lens correction. However, it has all but been abadoned.

(b) **Lamellar keratoplasty** retains the host endothelium, and graft rejection is reduced. It is a more demanding surgical procedure than penetrating keratoplasty and the optical results are often worse.

(c) **Penetrating keratoplasty** is undertaken when contact lens options are exhausted, particularly in patients who have significant corneal scarring. Results are usually excellent, as the peripheral cornea is essentially normal, and rejection is rare.

RGP lenses for keratoconus

If we were able to construct an ideal RGP patient, it is unlikely that he or she would bear much resemblance to the average keratoconic. Leaving aside the exotic corneal topograhy, the patient has a good chance of being atopic. Apart from the likelihood of allergic conjunctivitis for at least part of the year, the chances of solution sensitivity and of contact lens-related papillary conjunctivitis (CLPC) are higher. Then there are the personality traits. Anxiety, psychosomatic illness and a tendency to be somewhat "high maintenance" are all relatively common, as they are in other chronic eye diseases. On the credit side, keratoconic patients are often highly motivated, as contact lenses may be their only route to satisfactory vision. To summarize, we may be faced with a patient with a horrible cornea and multiple allergies who is very anxious to succeed, in every sense. The fitting process may be prolonged and involve a certain amount of improvisation on the part of the practitioner so it is important to manage expectations from the outset. This will reassure the patient when things appear to degenerate to trial and error, and may also be beneficial to the long-term mental health and blood pressure of the practitioner.

The fitting of patients with early keratoconus is likely to be similar to that for any astigmatic patient, but once the condition advances the corneal topography will require more specialized lenses. At one time, lenses were fitted with central bearing, in the hope of controlling disease progression. However, the effectiveness of this approach is controversial and there is now evidence (though at present not a huge amount) that this type of fit may initiate or exacerbate **corneal scarring**, so the desired goal now is to eliminate central bearing by fitting lenses with **apical clearance**. This is more easily arranged in early keratoconus and in many cases it is impossible to achieve. Alternatively, mid-peripheral bearing may relieve some of the pressure on the apex of the cone. This divided support, or **"three-point touch,"** is characterized by some central bearing with two mid-peripheral points, roughly 180° from each other, also bearing some of the weight. Mid-peripheral bearing may be impractical with the globus form of cone, and here large flat lenses may be the only option.

There are many designs available, though finding them in the ACLM manual is less easy than it might be. They are listed with conventional lenses, though the usual clue is the letter "K" in the title.

Aspheric lenses (e.g. Persecon E Keratoconus, CIBA) may work in early cases, and because peripheral plus power comes built in, early presbyopes may find these lenses useful. However, if they fail to center well the vision will be poor and optics based on spherical curves are more reliable. There are various designs available, of which the most popular in the UK are as follow.

The Soper Cone system uses bicurve lenses and the fitting philosophy is based on sagittal depth, using a combination of BOZRs and BOZDs. The fitting set consists of 10 lenses subdivided into "mild" (7.40 mm TD, 6.00 mm BOZD), "moderate" (8.50 mm TD, 7.00 mm BOZD) and "advanced" (9.50 mm TD, 8.00 mm BOZD) subsets. The aim is to avoid apical touch, but the bicurve construction may provide inadequate peripheral clearance which may cause the lens to seal off tear exchange.

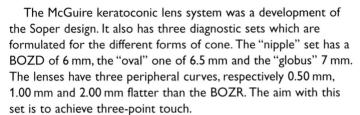

The McGuire keratoconic lens system was a development of the Soper design. It also has three diagnostic sets which are formulated for the different forms of cone. The "nipple" set has a BOZD of 6 mm, the "oval" one of 6.5 mm and the "globus" 7 mm. The lenses have three peripheral curves, respectively 0.50 mm, 1.00 mm and 2.00 mm flatter than the BOZR. The aim with this set is to achieve three-point touch.

The Rose K has complex, computer-generated peripheral curves based on several hundred fittings. The optic zone contracts as the base curve steepens. The aim is to achieve an ideal edge clearance 0.80 mm wide. The fitting set has standard edge lift, and after observation of the fluorescein pattern combinations can be selected which are 1.00, 1.50, 2.00, 2.50 or 3.00 mm flatter and 0.50 or 1.00 mm steeper than standard. BOZRs range from 4.75 to 8.00 and TDs from 7.90 to 10.20, and both front and back surface toricities are available. Some laboratories will supply this lens in Boston XO material which gives good oxygen permeability and the software used to generate the periphery makes this complex lens easily reproducible. Again, three-point touch is the aim.

Fitting protocol

There is a terrible old joke concerning a traveler lost in rural Ireland who encounters a farmer leaning on a gate. "Excuse me, my man, but how do I get to Dublin?" enquires the traveler. The farmer, after a long pause for deep cogitation, replies: "Well now, sir, I wouldn't start from here if I was you."

Before commencing the fitting of a keratoconic patient the more accurate information you have to hand, the quicker you are likely to arrive at a satisfactory outcome.

A current and accurate **spectacle Rx** is essential and by far the best way to ensure this is to do it yourself, even if the last refraction was recent. Keratoconics are difficult to refract accurately and somewhat variable. While it is always nice to have someone else to blame if things don't go to plan, it is better if they don't go wrong in the first place.

A topographical map is highly desirable to give an indication of the type of cone the patient has. Topographers often come with bundled software that can take the corneal data and custom design a lens for that cornea (e.g. Keratoconus [Wave] from Northern Lenses), often featuring simulated fluorescein patterns, or at least suggest a suitable trial lens to insert. In the absence of such sophisticated technology, fitting sets may be borrowed from manufacturers, and ideally more than one should be available to save time.

The **TD** and **BOZD** are selected by measuring the average pupil diameter and adding 1–2 mm, while ensuring that the optic zone fully covers the cone.

The **BOZR** is based on keratometry. The usual approach is to split the difference between steepest and flattest K readings, bearing in mind that these are not necessarily at 90° to each other. However, some practitioners advocate going rather steeper, aiming to insert an initial lens with apical clearance. By analyzing the fluorescein pattern, the BOZR can then be progressively flattened until apical touch is seen, and the final BOZR selected according to fitting philosophy. The changes in BOZR required to change the fluorescein pattern on a keratoconic cornea may be rather larger than those normally employed.

A drop of **anesthetic** inserted into the eye may help even with existing wearers, as excessive tearing will cause the lens to center poorly and make the fluorescein pattern difficult to interpret. The increased tear film may also cause over-minusing during over-refraction. It is worth giving a keratoconic patient half an hour or so for the lens to settle. The cone tends to be easily malleable so the fit may change.

The lens may need to be centered manually, using the lower lid, in order to correctly interpret the fit. Air bubbles may collect in the cone area. It is sometimes possible to reduce this by choosing a smaller BOZD. However, to retain sagittal depth the BOZR needs to be proportionally steeper.

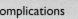

Keratoconus is a progressive condition and even established wearers will need to be seen every 6 months or so to ensure that the lenses are still fitting well. A number of issues may arise during aftercare:

1. **Staining** is common in keratoconus, and provided it is limited, does not necessarily require action. However, a whorl-shaped pattern, rather like a hurricane, may indicate restriction of tear flow under the lens due to excessive bearing. This type of staining sometimes precedes apical scarring.

2. **Lens associated scarring** begins as discrete nodules in Bowman's membrane which then increase in size and coalesce. It can occur within 3–4 months of contact lens wear. There may also be scarring which is not contact lens related. This can be in Bowman's but is often deeper in the stroma and may be circular or reticular.

3. **Solution reactions** are not uncommon, given that about half of all keratoconic patients may be atopic.

4. **Seal-off** of the periphery or mid-periphery may prevent adequate tear exchange and could cause lens binding. Any lens which rides low and doesn't move should be suspected of binding.

5. There tend to be **abnormal levels of deposits** and the complicated design of keratoconic lenses may make manual cleaning less efficient. In particular lenses with an anterior flange will often develop a ring deposit. Enzyme cleaners are probably going to be required.

6. **Hydrops** has been discussed on page 108. Patients will present with a white spot on the cornea and blurred vision.

7. **Poor vision** may be caused by a number of non-pathological causes:
    (a) **Over-minusing** at the time of fitting is common.

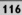
(b) **Lens flexure** may be reduced by using a thicker lens, though this will reduce oxygen transmission.
(c) **Residual astigmatism** may be present. It is always tempting to try to correct this with a bitoric design but on keratoconic patients this rarely works. Supplementary spectacles may be a better option visually.

Lens fitting after keratoplasty

At one time fitting was delayed until about a year after surgery, when all sutures had been removed. These days some at least of the sutures are left in indefinitely and only removed if complications occur. Lenses are often fitted 3–6 months after surgery. Occasionally, soft lenses may give a satisfactory result, but in most cases the irregular astigmatism induced requires some sort of rigid lens correction, which may take several forms:

1. Conventional RGP lens designs are sometimes successful.
2. Many post-keratoplasty corneas have a flattened central area requiring the use of modified or reverse geometry lenses similar to those used for orthokeratology. Topographical mapping of the cornea is essential to fit these lenses.
3. "Piggyback" fitting of an RGP lens on a soft lens, both lenses often specially modified, may help where lenses are reluctant to center.
4. Softperm lenses have a rigid optic zone with a hydrogel "skirt" and these have the same uses as piggyback designs.
5. Scleral lenses, by fitting the sclera and vaulting the cornea, make corneal geometry largely irrelevant. However, they require considerable skill and time to fit well and most scleral fitting is now done in a hospital or specialized practice setting.

8

Better sight without glasses: extended wear orthokeratology and fitting after refractive surgery

Introduction

As long as anyone can remember there have been those who yearn for the good vision that contact lenses will provide but without the inconvenience of maintaining them. By far the best way to achieve this is by a wise choice of parents, but for those less fortunate three strategies are available:

1. Extended wear contact lenses that correct the refractive error only for as long as the lenses are worn.
2. Orthokeratology which induces an actual (albeit temporary) change in refractive error.
3. Refractive surgery which produces a permanent change in refractive error.

Rigid contact lenses may be used for the first two strategies, and even after refractive surgery those with suboptimal outcomes may require a contact lens correction.

RGP extended wear

To most people, extended wear is associated with soft contact lenses of some sort, but rigid lenses have a rather longer history in this field. It is probable that contact lenses have been worn overnight by some patients, with or without the collusion of the practitioners who fitted them, for as long as contact lenses have been in existence. Some of the early glass haptic lenses fitted in the 1880s are known to have been worn continuously for up to 2 years at a time. Many adventurous souls have experimented since with both haptics and PMMA corneal lenses, with or without the connivance, or indeed awareness, of their practitioners. The introduction of gas-permeable materials in the 1970s made the use of rigid lenses for extended wear a more viable proposition and their use increased gradually in the 1980s. Fewer adverse responses and localized physiological responses were reported with RGPs than with the hydrogel materials also in use for extended wear. By the end of the 1980s concern was rising on the incidence of microbial keratitis in extended wear patients, and while the majority of papers suggested that soft extended wear was the major concern, the ensuing publicity all but killed off the extended wear market for all lens types.

The bubble burst in 1989 with the publication of a study by Poggio and Schein. Extended wear patients were found to have an incidence of keratitis of 20.9 per 100 000 patients compared to 4.1 per 100 000 in patients wearing hydrogel lenses on a daily basis. In 1989 the FDA recommended that extended wear be limited to less than 7 days and 6 nights before removal, although the US contact lens industry had already taken this step voluntarily.

More recently, silicone hydrogel lenses have received approval for extended wear up to 30 days in the UK. The research that accompanied their development suggested that chronic hypoxia played a major role in the association of extended wear with microbial keratitis; however, recent studies have suggested that hypoxia is only one of a number of issues, albeit an important one. There has also been a revival of interest in orthokeratology using high Dk RGP lenses worn overnight. Most RGP lenses are worn up to a maximum of 7 days, but the emergence of a "hyper-Dk" RGP material has raised the possibility of wear up to 30 days.

Advantages and disadvantages of extended wear

Most extended wear is elective and offers no particular clinical advantage over other modalities save that of convenience. However, there are some clinical advantages for certain patients:

1. Handling is kept to a minimum. It is probable that a significant proportion of the physical abrasions that the cornea suffers occur during insertion and removal. The elderly, physically impaired or very young patient may be safer with a lens that requires little or no handling.

2. Compliance with solution regimes is largely eliminated, although we are still reliant on the patient to remove, clean and disinfect the lenses at specified intervals.

3. Some patients, admittedly a minority, are somewhat heavy-handed when cleaning their lenses. A vice-like grip and rough skin may cause the lens surface to deteriorate rapidly when cleaned daily.

4. The demands of certain careers might compromise the safety of the wearer, or of others, if lengthy cleaning and disinfection procedures have to be undertaken daily. Members of the armed forces and emergency services fall into this group.

5. Occasionally, low vision practitioners attempt to create a Galilean telescope using a high-powered negative contact lens with a high positive spectacle lens. Patients who would find this useful will find handling of a small contact lens challenging.

However, extended wear does present a greater physiological challenge to the eye, and this is reflected in the greater incidence of inflammatory events, including microbial keratitis (MK), associated with this modality. For RGP lenses studies have suggested an approximately threefold increase in MK when the lenses are worn on an extended wear basis. The exact incidence is difficult to pin down as the precise criteria for MK vary from study to study, but for extended wear figures between 4.2 and 18.2 per 10 000 wearers annually have been published.

Advantages and disadvantages of RGP extended wear

Modern RGP lenses have considerable advantages over hydrogel materials and are a viable alternative to silicone hydrogel lenses. The advantages of RGP lenses in extended wear include:

1. High oxygen permeability, giving oxygen flux readings comparable to silicone hydrogels.

2. The lenses are smaller than the soft equivalent so they cover less of the cornea, which also aids oxygen provision and reduces the incidence of neovascularization.

3. The presence of an active tear pump supplements the oxygen supply through tear exchange under the lens.
4. Lens mobility and tear exchange will aid the flushing of debris and microorganisms from beneath the lens, which should in theory reduce the incidence of certain inflammatory events. In a recent trial of hyper-Dk materials, a lower incidence of infiltrates was found with 30-day RGP wear than with 7-day wear with a hydrogel material.
5. The lens material may deposit less, dehydrate less and have a longer life than soft materials.
6. Visual quality is often better with rigid lenses. Until recently extended wear for those patients with significant astigmatism was only feasible with RGP lenses; however, toric silicone hydrogels are now available. Patients with irregular corneas will only achieve satisfactory vision with a rigid lens.
7. Compared with hydrogel materials, though perhaps not silicone hydrogels, RGPs show significantly lower risk of infection, even in the presence of contraindicative factors such as smoking and blepharitis. Very high Dk RGP materials also resist adherence by *Pseudomonas aeruginosa*, even in extended wear conditions.

Chronic hypoxia and the cornea

During waking hours the cornea receives its oxygen supply from the atmosphere. When the eyes are closed, oxygen is supplied almost exclusively from the capillary plexus of the palpebral conjunctiva, and the level of oxygen available is approximately one-third of that available when the eyes are open. Without adequate oxygen the corneal epithelium responds with anaerobic metabolic activity. This results in a build-up of lactic acid which in turn osmotically induces the influx of fluid into the corneal stroma, resulting in edema. The situation is made worse by the increase in temperature behind the closed lids which speeds up metabolic processes, creating a greater oxygen demand. Even without contact lens wear the average cornea swells by some 4% during sleep but can recover when the eye opens. About 8% of swelling can be recovered during the day.

The development of silicone hydrogels has provided a great deal of information on the effects of hypoxia on corneal integrity. The main effects are seen at the three levels that contain cells:

1. The **epithelium** will show reduced cell mitosis and cell migration, and a loss of tight junctions. The result is a thinner barrier that is more easily damaged mechanically and will repair more slowly. This in turn will provide a greater opportunity for microbial infection.
2. The **stroma** will initially swell as a result of the intake of water caused by the epithelium and endothelium being less able to pump it out. A build-up of carbon dioxide (hypercapnia) leads to a fall in pH (acidosis) and this can lead in time to keratocyte death, with subsequent thinning of the stroma.
3. The **endothelium** will often show signs of distress, although it is not known to what extent its function is compromised. Reduction in cell count and variations in the apparent size and shape of the cells may be detected with the major slit-lamp. Some of these changes may not be reversible.

In addition, bacterial adherence to corneal tissue appears to be greater in hypoxic conditions.

The presence of a contact lens will further reduce the availability of oxygen to the cornea. The degree to which it does this will depend how quickly the oxygen can traverse the lens. In addition, the tonicity of the tears will fall somewhat, facilitating the influx of fluid into the cornea, and RGP lenses have a greater effect than soft ones.

In 1984, Holden and Mertz found that a level of Dk/t of 87×10^9 Fatt units was required to give less than 4% edema in overnight wear. It should be stressed that this is an average figure, and that there appears to be considerable individual variation. That said, a number of RGP and silicone hydrogel materials appear to fulfill the Holden–Mertz criteria for extended wear. However, Dk/t may not be the best way to compare oxygen availability. Several researchers have advocated the use of oxygen flux as a measure of the volume of oxygen transmitted over time.

Many RGP materials offer comparable performance to silicone hydrogels.

Recently, a lens with very high oxygen transmission has appeared, and this has received FDA approval for extended wear up to 30 days. The Menicon Z (Menicon) is a fluoromethacrylate lens that incorporates a novel siloxanylstyrene monomer. This allows improved stability at high Dk and a low affinity for lipid deposits. The reported Dk is 163, which should place it well above the Holden–Mertz criterion. Initial clinical findings with the lens have been encouraging and it would seem to offer a viable alternative to silicone hydrogel lenses for those seeking extended wear.

Fitting RGP extended wear lenses

The characteristics of a good extended wear lens are essentially the same as those of any other RGP lens. There is a trend towards using topographical data to achieve closer corneal alignment (as in the Z-wave system) and towards larger total diameters (10–11 mm being typical). Both measures are intended to improve comfort, but those very characteristics which make an RGP lens comfortable are also those which make it prone to binding, so a degree of compromise may be required.

Successful daily wear of RGP lenses is a prerequisite of RGP extended wear, and several aftercare visits may be required before overnight wear is attempted. Patients should be seen after the first night of extended wear, preferably in the morning when clinical signs may be more apparent. Subsequent appointments are typically after 3 and 7 days of extended wear, then after a month and at intervals of 3–6 months for as long as the patient continues with lens wear.

It should be stressed that even if the lenses are capable of supporting 30 days of continuous wear, shorter periods may reduce the incidence of adverse effects.

Every morning the patient should be encouraged to carry out a self-assessment of the lens by asking:

1. Do the eyes look good? (i.e. are they white – hyperemia is not a normal sign with these lenses).

2. Do they feel good? Are the lenses moving well? If not an ocular lubricant may help. Lens movement is essential to flush debris from beneath the lens and an immobile lens is likely to cause an inflammatory reaction, or worse.

3. Can I see well? Check each eye in turn.

If the answer to any of these questions is no, the wearer should remove the lenses and contact their practitioner as soon as possible. Emergency contact procedures should be established and recorded. Printed agreements signed by both the practitioner and patient may prevent undue and erroneous claims in the event of a major concern in the future.

Orthokeratology

Orthokeratology is a process in which rigid contact lenses are used to induce changes in corneal curvature, thereby modifying refractive error. The cornea is easily deformed by external pressure. Indeed, this is the basis of applanation tonometry. PMMA contact lenses also regularly produced changes in corneal curvature and refractive error but this was generally seen as a side-effect, and not a particularly desirable one. In 1962, Jessen suggested that these changes could be used deliberately to modify refractive error. For the rest of the 1960s and 70s a number of practitioners attempted to put this idea into practice but results were variable. Each practitioner used a different lens design or replacement schedule and properly controlled experimental data were thin on the ground. The other major problem was that the refractive changes were not permanent. Once lens wear ceased, regression began.

Orthokeratology has continued to be a minority interest, but a number of developments have re-stimulated interest in recent years. Possibly the most significant development has been the emergence of videokeratography, allowing detailed topographical analysis of the whole cornea. Lenses can be designed more precisely for individual corneas and induced changes observed in much greater detail, which in turn will lead to better design algorithms for the lenses.

Orthokeratology took a large step forward with the introduction of **reverse geometry lenses**. Early orthokeratology lenses tended to be large and flat, and they often didn't center well. This in turn could lead to induced astigmatism, the opposite effect to the one expected. Reverse geometry lenses have a flat central base curve with a steeper secondary curve. They center better even when the central curve is considerably flatter than the cornea and the steeper secondary curve. These lenses can achieve more rapid change than the old designs, so use of them is sometimes termed "accelerated orthokeratology."

There is some evidence that reverse geometry lenses do a little more than simple flattening of the central cornea. Swarbrick et al (1998) found a number of changes:

1. Flattening of the central cornea.
2. Central corneal thinning, probably mostly epithelial.
3. Mid-peripheral corneal thickening, mostly stromal.

The results suggest that orthokeratology is not just a simple process of bending the cornea. Tissue redistribution may also be taking place, possibly in response to the pressure exerted by the tear reservoir under the lens. Of course, if this is true, more conventional lenses could also induce tissue redistribution in various patterns, but as yet there are no data.

Will it work?

The effects of the earlier designs were varied. Some practitioners claimed to have corrected 4–5.00D of myopia but most claimed considerably less. More recent studies using reverse geometry lenses seem to agree that the average change expected would be 1.50D ± 0.50D and about half of the corneal astigmatism is eliminated. There is significant individual variability. For higher refractive errors it is unlikely to be a complete solution on its own.

Predicting success is a challenge. High myopes tend to change less than those with mid-range prescriptions. It is claimed that corneal asphericity is an important determinant of success. Most corneas flatten towards the periphery and are said to have a positive shape factor. During orthokeratology, the cornea flattens more centrally than peripherally, to the point where the shape factor is effectively zero and the cornea more or less spherical. At this point, no further flattening is likely. Mountford (1997) found a direct correlation between corneal shape and induced change.

The importance of corneal shape factor makes videokeratography an essential tool for this type of practice. It has long been known that the refractive changes measured by subjective refraction are often rather larger than those predicted by keratometry. Swarbrick et al (1998) found that the changes in curvature are most marked in the center of the cornea, diminishing towards the periphery. Keratometry measures corneal curvature some way off the center, so will never detect the full extent of the induced changes.

Regression

The induced changes in corneal curvature are not permanent. As soon as contact lens wear is suspended the corneal change, and thus the refractive error, begins to regress. The rate of regression varies but the typical value is 0.50D per day. In order to sustain the new refractive status some wearing of contact lenses is essential. These **"retainer"** or **"sleeper"** lenses may be worn during the day or overnight.

Night therapy

The availability of high-transmission materials has made it possible to wear the orthokeratology lenses overnight and remove them for the day. Patients whose occupations require a specified level of unaided vision may find this option useful, as may the terminally vain. The lenses must be treated in the same way as any other lens worn overnight. The design of reverse geometry lenses may contribute towards a tendency to adhere to the cornea, and lenses are now being designed to fit a little looser in an attempt to overcome this problem.

Is it safe?

On the evidence so far there seems to be no greater risk with modern orthokeratology lenses than with conventional RGP lenses in a similar wearing modality. Complications do occur, but only at the same rate and of the same type as those of RGP wearers generally. The long-term effects of central epithelial thinning remain to be seen. In addition, the possible link between eye-rubbing, RGP wear and keratoconus suggests that placing repeated pressure on the cornea may not be an entirely good idea for some patients, and for many practitioners the jury is still out.

Initial lens selection

Conventional orthokeratology lenses

These lenses are generally multicurve designs fitted initially 0.50 mm flatter than K. Lid attachment is essential, both to enable the lens to center and because upper lid pressure is a major source of the force that modifies the cornea. Centration is important as a poorly centered lens may induce astigmatism.

Reverse geometry lenses

The initial central base curve is selected 1.00–2.00D (0.20–0.40 mm) flatter than flattest K though the secondary curve will be considerably steeper. A small BOZD will tend to maximize the orthokeratology effect, as the smaller sag will produce a flatter fitting relationship with the cornea. However, a larger BOZD may be required in order for the lens to center well, or by a large pupil. The larger the BOZD, the flatter the BOZR required. A trial fitting set saves a lot of time at this stage.

The fluorescein pattern required should show moderate apical bearing over the central 3–5 mm, then an annulus of mid-peripheral pooling about 2 mm wide. Edge clearance must be adequate to allow good tear exchange and prevent "sealing-off," especially if overnight wear is envisaged. Once the fit is satisfactory, over-refraction will determine the power required.

Subsequent care

The care of orthokeratology lenses is the same as conventional ones. It is worth seeing conventional orthokeratology patients 1 week after collection to check progress. With reverse geometry lenses, the effects may be quicker and a first aftercare examination may be required sooner. An initial check after 3–4 hours' wear on the day of collection may help to set this interval. The intervals for subsequent visits will depend on the rate of change, which tends to slow after the first couple of weeks. Once the change grinds to a halt, going flatter may yield further rewards. It is worth ordering more than one pair of lenses, with BOZRs flatter at intervals of 0.50–1.00 mm flatter than the first pair. If the cornea changes rapidly, the fit of the lenses may become inappropriate and it is useful to have the remedy to hand.

The ultimate aim should be a residual spectacle refraction of about +0.50 or so, which should allow distance visual acuity to be maintained during the day.

However, it may not be possible to achieve this endpoint, so patient expectations must be managed carefully. Once further change is impractical, some contact lens wear will be required to maintain the new refractive status. The exact amount will depend on the patient and a certain amount of experimentation may be necessary. The retainer lens is usually the last orthokeratology lens used provided the fit is adequate. Overnight wear may be possible with appropriate lenses. Regular aftercare (every 3–6 months) is necessary, even for patients on retainer wear.

Orthokeratology is labor-intensive compared to more normal contact lens practice. Diagnostic fitting is normally required, and access to a videokeratoscope more or less essential. Frequent aftercare visits are involved. For this reason, it can never be done cheaply and a realistic fee structure is essential. With accelerated orthokeratology, a further challenge may be the short interval between appointments which can be difficult to accommodate in a busy optometric practice.

The future?

The difficulty in predicting the future in a book is that by the time people read the prediction it's probably history. At present, some degree of success is being obtained in hyperopic cases in addition to the more usual myopes. **Corneaplasty** has also been trialled in which an enzyme is injected into the corneal stroma which weakens the molecular bonds holding the collagen fibrils together. The resultant softer cornea is then reshaped in the usual way, then injected with a second solution that reverses the effect of the first. The idea is that the cornea will retain the new profile, eliminating the need for retainer lenses. Practitioner enthusiasm at this time is mixed.

Fitting contact lenses following refractive surgery

Refractive surgery has been with us now for half a century and while constant improvement in patient selection protocols and surgical techniques has occurred, there has inevitably been the odd occasion when things have not gone entirely to plan. In the UK, approximately 75 000 procedures were undertaken in 2001 and this probably doubled in 2002, but the market for refractive surgery appears to have leveled out for the moment. There have been numerous surgical techniques applied to the modification of refractive error and it is beyond the scope of this volume to cover them in any detail. We will concentrate on those patients an optometrist in general practice is most likely to encounter, either as a new fitting or an existing contact lens wearer.

1. **RK** (radial keratotomy) involves the placing of a number of radial incisions in the mid-periphery of the cornea. The wounds created gape open and are filled initially with an epithelial plug, and eventually with fibroplastic scar tissue. This has the effect of flattening the cornea over most of its surface, but more so in the central area. The result is a shift in refractive error towards hyperopia. The degree of flattening obtained depends on the number, depth and length of the incisions, and also on individual variation in the wound-healing process. In some patients the radial scars may be raised above the corneal surface, and this can cause decentration of a rigid lens as the raised areas act as pivot points. The scars are also prone to neovascularization.

2. **PRK** (photorefractive keratotomy) and its variants have largely but not entirely supplanted RK. This involves the use of an excimer laser to ablate the corneal stroma after the epithelium is removed by photoablation or scraping. In **LASIK** (laser in situ keratomilieusis, "flap and zap"), a microkeratome is used to cut a flap of epithelium and underlying anterior stroma which is replaced onto the ablated stromal bed. This procedure is less painful to the patient and recovery is quicker. **LASEK** (laser epithelial keratomileusis) is similar to PRK but an epithelial flap is created which is replaced after ablation. Between 95 and 98% of patients will achieve a satisfactory outcome, but the remainder may need an alternative form of optical correction as further surgery may be impractical or undesirable.

Patients who require contact lenses after undergoing refractive surgery may not be ideal contact lens candidates. They can be rather demanding individuals, with a perfectionist streak that may have motivated them to seek surgery in the first place. They may be less than enthused about having to wear contact lenses, because if they had been that keen on the idea they would not have had the surgery. They will probably be even less keen on spectacle wear, and so likely to demand (sometimes literally) long wearing times or even extended wear. The failure of their expensive refractive surgery may also have colored their perception of eye care professionals in general, and not in a good way. Finally the surgical process may have left a physiological legacy which complicates the fitting process:

1. In rare cases, too much corneal tissue may be removed, or the patient may have had undetected keratoconus forme fruste. The result is **keratectasia,** in which the cornea protrudes in a way similar to keratoconus. Management is essentially the same as for keratoconus.
2. Irregular astigmatism may be induced by a decentered ablation zone or flap displacement. It can also occur if there is epithelial ingrowth under the flap, or inflammation of the interface (known variously as diffuse lamellar keratitis, DLK, or "sands of the Sahara").
3. Corneal sensitivity is reduced following LASIK and PRK as corneal nerves are cut or destroyed. After PRK, recovery to nearly normal levels occurs after about a month, whereas after LASIK recovery takes 3–6 months, and post-surgery corneas do not appear to ever quite return to full sensitivity. The reduced sensitivity can affect the blink reflex and slow epithelial wound healing.
4. A further consequence of reduced corneal sensitivity is reduced tear production, which may persist for 9 months after surgery, and dry eye symptoms are very common among post-surgical patients.
5. The cornea will have altered topography. After surgery to reduce myopia, the cornea becomes "oblate," i.e. flatter in the center than the periphery, whereas after the less common correction of hyperopia the central cornea will be steeper than before.

The amount of corneal tissue ablated will largely determine the types of contact lens that can be fitted. The **Munnerlyn formula** gives the depth of ablation for a given refractive correction and optic zone.

$$\text{Depth of ablation} \atop \text{(microns)} = \frac{(\text{optic zone diameter})^2 \times (\text{refractive error})}{3}$$

When less than 50 microns has been removed rigid and soft lenses of conventional geometry will generally work, so for corrections of up to about 4.00D postoperative fitting should be fairly straightforward. However, higher refractive change will remove more tissue and the difference in curvature between central and mid-peripheral areas requires reverse geometry lenses similar to those used for orthokeratology and post-keratoplasty lenses.

When fitting a post-surgical cornea there is a dilemma over what measurements to base the initial selection of the lens parameters on. In general, fairly large total diameters are used, so that the lens edge avoids the flap perimeter. If the preoperative K readings are used there is likely to be a fair bit of central clearance. There will be a thick, positive tear film that will require extra minus power to correct. If the postoperative Ks are consulted the central fit will be better, but the lens is likely to have excessive edge clearance and be somewhat uncomfortable. You could split the difference between the two sets of readings, or take the K reading 4 mm temporarily, but whatever the starting point there may need to be some independent adjustment of the central and peripheral curves. Topographical mapping is extremely helpful and refractive surgery clinics will often supply these data if requested.

Reverse geometry lenses may be ordered after using appropriate fitting sets, or by fitting the optic and peripheral zones separately with conventional lenses. Alternatively, if topographical data are sent to the laboratory, lenses can be custom designed for that individual cornea.

References

Holden BA, Mertz GW (1984) Critical oxygen levels to avoid corneal oedema for daily and extended wear. *Invest. Ophthal. Vis. Sci.* **25**:1161–7.

Jessen GN (1962) Orthofocus techniques. *Contacto* **6**:200–4.

Mountford JA (1997) Orthokeratology. In *Contact Lenses*, 4th edn (ed. Phillips AJ & Speedwell L) pp. 653–92. Butterworth-Heinemann, Oxford.

Poggio EG, Schein OD (1989) The incidence of ulcerative keratitis among wearers of daily wear and extended wear soft contact lenses. *N. Engl. J. Med.* **321**:779–83.

Swarbrick HA, Wong G, O'Leary DJ (1998) Corneal response to orthokeratology. *Optom. Vis. Sci.* **75**:791–9.

9
Collection and lens care

Introduction

The advice given at the collection (or "teach") appointment is an important factor in the success or failure of any contact lens wear. Collection is often delegated to unqualified staff, but it remains the responsibility of the prescribing practitioner to ensure that the advice given is both sound and safe.

During this appointment the patient must be educated in the following areas:

1. The importance of hygiene.
2. Safe insertion and removal of the lenses.
3. Adaptation schedule.
4. How to recognize when things are going wrong.
5. The importance of regular aftercare and the probable consequences of non-compliance.
6. Correct use of their care regime.

Hygiene

Fingers that insert contact lenses need to have short fingernails to minimize the risk to the cornea. Patients with long nails should be advised to cut them short, and the time to do this is before the lenses are fitted. Careful hand-washing is essential before handling lenses, and the practitioner should set a good example during the initial fitting process and check during aftercare appointments that the patient has not forgotten this important step.

Insertion and removal of lenses

In order to insert a contact lens, the patient must override their own ocular defense mechanisms, and some find this easier than others. In general women find this a little easier, provided they have experience in applying eye make-up, but there are exceptions. In some cases a dry run without lenses may help to overcome any squeamishness.

The lens should always be inspected before insertion to ensure that it has no damage or debris attached. Sufficient conditioning solution should be spread over the lens surface to enable the lens to adhere to the patient's finger in any position, but it is counterproductive to fill the "bowl" of the lens with solution as this merely adds extra weight to the lens, which will probably end up on the floor. The lens is placed on the tip of either the first or the middle finger of the right hand (to insert the right lens) (Figure 9.1), depending on patient preference.

It helps if the applying fingertip is as dry as possible before placing the lens ("dry finger, wet lens"), and dabbing it on a lint-free tissue before picking up the lens may help the lens to transfer to the eye.

To insert the right lens, the patient is instructed to look down. The left hand is brought to rest on the forehead and the tip of the middle finger is placed on the upper lid margin of the right

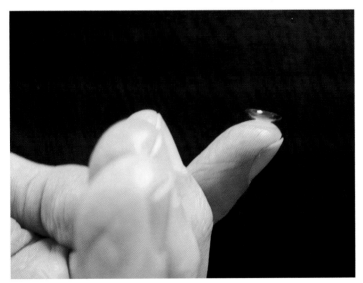

Figure 9.1   Lens is placed on finger ready for insertion

eye next to the lashes. The lid is pulled up, and provided the placement of the finger is correct, the patient should be unable to blink with the finger in place (Figure 9.2).

The patient is then instructed to look into a mirror. The lower lid is gently pulled down by the tip of either the middle or the ring finger of the right hand, depending which feels more comfortable to the patient. The lens is then applied to the cornea, with the patient encouraged to maintain fixation on their eye in the mirror so as to counteract Bell's phenomenon. The patient should then ensure that the lens is correctly centered on the cornea by checking whether they can see with that eye.

New wearers tend to approach the eye with the lens at a snail's pace, which gives them more opportunity to lose their nerve, and they have a tendency to let go of the lids and look away from the mirror at the moment of insertion. Gentle coaching is required to overcome this, and patience is a considerable virtue here. Should the lens come to rest on the

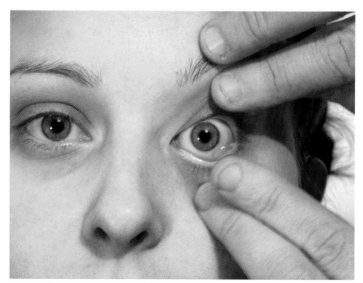

Figure 9.2   Lids held ready for insertion

sclera, the patient should be shown how to use the eyelids to move the lens to the temporal sclera for removal, rather than attempting to re-center the lens. It is worth showing every new lens wearer how to do this, as there will eventually come a time when every patient will miss the cornea.

Removal of the lens can be achieved by either the "pull and blink" technique or the "pinch" technique detailed in Chapter 4. The optimal method may depend on the individual. The patient should fixate their own eye in the mirror with the head turned slightly to the same side as the eye from which the lens is being removed (Figure 9.3).

Removal may be easier if the mirror is placed flat on the desk with the patient looking down. This should ensure that the lid forces act equally on the lens and expel it, rather than send it sideways. Once the patient has got the hang of this, those using the pull and blink method should be encouraged to bring the other hand close to the eye so as to catch the lens as it exits the eye.

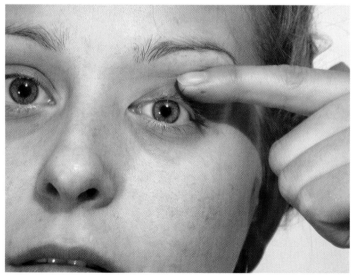

Figure 9.3 Patient using "pull and blink" method of removal

New patients should be observed inserting and removing their lenses at least three times. Established wearers should be observed at least once to ensure that their technique is safe. Occasionally, they may need to be re-educated.

Adaptation schedule

The patient must adapt to the lid sensation that the lens edges will impart, and the cornea to the physiological challenge of the lens, so a gradual increase in wearing time is helpful. Typically, the patient is instructed to wear the lens for 2 hours on the first day and add an extra 2 hours a day subsequently. Some practitioners speed things up by recommending wear in the morning followed by a break in the afternoon and reinserting the lenses in the evening, but this should be judged on an individual basis.

Provided the instruction on handling has not left the patient with too much trauma (and it is wise to check) it will boost confidence if the patient can leave the practice wearing the lenses. However, sometimes new lenses do not wet particularly well, particularly if delivered in a dry state, and storage of the lenses for 24 hours may help.

Recognizing normal and abnormal

It is important that the patient should be able to tell the difference between the normal symptoms that accompany adaptation to rigid lenses and those circumstances that require intervention. Mild foreign body sensation and intermittent blurring is to be expected initially, but it should reduce over the first few days. Significant redness and/or pain, especially if persistent after lens removal, should be recognized as abnormal. The patient should be advised to suspend lens wear and contact the practitioner promptly.

Reduction in vision should elicit a similar response, though it might be worth checking whether the lenses are in the correct eyes before calling out the cavalry. Most patients have managed to mix up their lenses at some time, and one of the authors once managed to drive to work with both lenses in the same eye.

The UK Opticians Act 1989 (Amendment) Order obliges the last practitioner to participate in the fitting of the lenses to provide:

1. A signed, written specification of the lenses fitted.
2. Instructions and information on the care, wear, treatment, cleaning and maintenance of the lens.

The specification should be issued once you are satisfied with the lens. This would normally be after the first aftercare appointment. The instructions on lens care must be issued at the time of collection.

Patients need to be aware of the possible consequences of poor lens care, and should have the opportunity to ask questions. It is worth reinforcing verbal instructions with written information, as much of the former may be forgotten. Most practitioners issue a standard consent form which is signed by the patient (or guardian in the case of a minor) to acknowledge that the proper advice and instructions have been given. One copy should be kept with the clinical records and one issued to the patient. The exact legal status of such declarations has never been tested in a British court, but it is better than nothing.

Aftercare

The new regulations place the practitioner under a duty to "make arrangements" for the wearer to receive aftercare but without actually defining aftercare. This obligation applies in circumstances and over a time period which is reasonable in a particular case, but the patient should not leave the practice with lenses unless an aftercare schedule has been discussed and the first appointment preferably booked. It is customary to see the patient 1–2 weeks after collection, but individual patients may require other intervals.

Care regimes

Until the 1990s, the care of PMMA and RGP lenses changed very little. There were often separate solutions for wetting, storage and cleaning, and in the case of RGP lenses this might be supplemented by the use of enzyme cleaners to remove protein. The complexity of such systems was never a help to encourage patient compliance, and the preservatives then in common use were inclined to give rise to toxic and allergic reactions. In an attempt to avoid these, and to address the changing characteristics of new lens materials, a new generation of care systems has superseded the previous one, and it is the newer systems that we will concentrate on now.

Rigid lenses require solutions to fulfill the following functions:

1. Cushioning the lens on insertion and allowing the lens to wet efficiently ("conditioning").
2. Cleaning.
3. Disinfection.

Conditioning is achieved by the incorporation of wetting agents. The most common are the following:

1. PVA (polyvinyl alcohol) has both lipophilic and hydrophilic groups. The former are attracted to the lens surface and the latter attract water, enabling the lens to wet.
2. Methylcellulose adds more viscosity than PVA. This will improve the cushioning effect but it may take a little longer for the vision to settle after insertion. Unfortunately methylcellulose, unlike PVA, can inhibit epithelial regeneration.

Buffering agents may be added to the solution to maintain a stable pH and promote lens comfort.

Daily cleaning is essential. The preservatives contained within contact lens solutions are designed to work on clean lenses and may be ineffective on lenses that are not cleaned first.

The most efficient cleaners are separate from the conditioning and storage solution, but a number of multipurpose products are available which are intended to fulfill both functions. Cleaning agents work in the following ways:

1. **Surfactant cleaners** remove contaminants in a way analogous to the effect of washing-up liquid on a plate. A common example is LC-65 (Allergan).
2. **Abrasive cleaners** shear deposits from the surface. Particles are incorporated to increase the abrasive effect of rubbing on the lens. Opti-free daily cleaner (AMO) uses polymeric beads. Boston Advance cleaner has small particles which are intended to preserve the high polish of FSA lenses. There is also a non-ionic surfactant incorporated that is aimed at the lipid deposits to which FSAs are prone. Abrasive cleaners may cause scratching of the lens or even an increase in minus power with heavy-handed use. However, few patients are this enthusiastic with regard to cleaning their lenses.
3. **Benzyl alcohol** may be combined with a surfactant to combat biofilms. *Pseudomonas aeruginosa* and *Serratia marcescens* produce biofilms that bind the bacteria into a colony and protect it from chemical attack.

Effective daily cleaning and rinsing of lenses probably accounts for 90% or more of the disinfection process as well as removing tear components which could otherwise cause toxic or allergic reactions and poor wetting if they were allowed to remain on the lens. Cleaning should be carried out immediately upon lens removal, though many patients will do this the following morning, if at all, when left to their own devices. The "morning-after method" has the twin disadvantages of rendering the preservatives in the storage solution impotent and ensuring that there will be residual cleaning agents on the lens when it is inserted. The correct procedure for cleaning the lens should be demonstrated to the patient:

1. The lens is placed in the palm of the hand with 2–3 drops of cleaning solution and rubbed for about 20 seconds on each

side, using a finger in a circular motion. Cleaning between the fingers may cause warpage.

2. The lens is rinsed with storage solution and placed in **fresh** (not recycled or topped-up) storage solution in the case.

Rigid lenses generally have much longer working life than soft ones, and it may become necessary to supplement daily cleaning with one of the **protein removal systems** originally developed for soft lenses. New lenses rarely need such systems, particularly those made from FSA or hybrid materials, but as the lenses become abraded with use the level of deposits of all kinds tends to increase. The frequency of use of these systems will vary according to the lens material and the tear chemistry of the individual patient, but typically it ranges from monthly to weekly. Consideration should be given to the rather better strategy of planned replacement of the lens to prevent it reaching the state where frequent protein removal is necessary.

It is important to recognize the difference between **disinfection** and **sterilization**. The former implies that all active pathogens have been neutralized, whereas the latter involves the elimination of inactive forms (e.g. *Acanthamoeba* cysts) as well. Rigid lenses are unlikely ever to be sterile and even disinfection may be a goal rather than a frequently obtained state, given that contact lens patients are rarely ideally compliant. However, careful use of the solutions should minimize the risk of infection. Historically, rigid lenses were disinfected with chemicals such as benzalkonium chloride, thimerosal and chlorhexidine gluconate but these had a tendency to cause sensitivity reactions. The first two have largely been supplanted, but chlorhexidine is still used, albeit at lower concentrations. Most solutions now contain polyhexanide or similar large-molecule preservatives (e.g. Polyquad) either singly or in combination with chlorhexidine.

1. **Chlorhexidine gluconate** is used in Boston Advance and Bausch & Lomb Elite in conjunction with hydrophilic components to discourage binding to the lens surface. It is effective against bacteria but has limited action against yeasts and fungi. Generally it is used in conjunction with polyhexanide.

2. **Polyhexanide** belongs to the same chemical family as chlorhexidene but has a larger molecular weight. It is attracted towards the negatively charged surface of the bacterial cell and subsequently disrupts cell membrane activity. It has a greater effectivity than chlorhexidine against *Serratia marcescens*, which secretes exotoxins capable of irritating the eye and stimulating mucus secretion.
3. **EDTA** is a chelating agent that removes calcium ions. This assists both cleaning and disinfection.

The use of **tap water** used to be commonplace among rigid lens wearers, but it should be remembered that the domestic water supply has been identified as source of *Acanthamoeba* contamination. RGP wearers are not immune to *Acanthamoeba* infection, and *Acanthamoeba* may find it easier to adhere to a rigid lens than to a soft one. For this reason tap water should not come into contact with the lenses, or indeed the case. Case contamination can be minimized by rinsing out the lens with solution or saline and air-drying, then replacing with fresh solution daily. Ideally, the case should be scrubbed weekly with a toothbrush, though few patients seem to keep this up for long after initial collection. Fortunately, many solutions now come packaged with a new case, but even then patients may need to be encouraged to use the new one. Cases that are used for too long will accumulate biofilm and may constitute a serious risk of infection. When surveys have been conducted on contact lens cases in the past, a majority have been found to be contaminated with one or more unpleasant microbes.

Re-use of rigid trial lenses

In 1999, the Spongiform Encephalopathy Advisory Committee (SEAC) advised the Department of Health of a remote theoretical risk of the transmission of prion protein associated with variant Creutzfeldt–Jakob disease (vCJD) by contact lenses or other devices which contact the eye, such as tonometer heads. Variant CJD is a progressive and fatal condition affecting the central nervous system. As a result, the College of Optometrists and the Association of Dispensing Opticians were asked to provide clinical guidelines to restrict contact lenses and optical devices to single patient use wherever practical, and suitable protocols for the cleaning of such devices where single use was impractical. **In general, lenses should be used on only one patient**, after which the lens is dispensed to that patient or disposed of by the practitioner. **Special complex diagnostic contact lenses** are defined as lenses used by a clinician to assess performance of a design on the eye. In general this is only applicable where there is disease or abnormality of the lid, cornea or ocular surface and most instances would therefore arise in hospital practice. However, use by university departments for training purposes is also permitted.

If re-use of lenses is undertaken the following conditions should be observed:

1. The lenses should be used solely within the clinician's premises and under the control of the clinician at all times.
2. The clinician should ensure that decontamination is carried out to the highest possible standards.
3. The clinician should keep full records to show the usage of each lens.
4. The clinician should inform the patient of all the relevant risks and benefits associated with contact lens fitting. It is best practice to obtain the patient's signature on an acknowledgment form. A suitable form of words is to be found in the Department of Health publication *Contact Lenses and You*.

Certain categories of patient should only be fitted with single-use lenses because of an increased risk of vCJD:

1. Recipients of pituitary derived hormones such as human growth hormone or gonadotrophins.
2. People known or assumed to have had human dura mater implanted, including people who have had brain surgery before

August 1982, and people who have had an operation for a tumor or a cyst of the spine before August 1992.
3. People diagnosed or suspected of suffering from CJD of any type, or with a family history of CJD.
4. People with degenerative neurological diseases of unknown causation.

Following use of the contact lens, the following procedure should be used:

1. The item to be decontaminated should not be allowed to dry following use.
2. It should be cleaned in the usual manner.
3. It should then be soaked in 2% sodium hypochlorite solution (readily available for domestic use) for 1 hour.
4. It should be removed from the solution and residual solution shaken off.
5. It should be thoroughly rinsed with sterile normal saline solution or freshly boiled water at room temperature.
6. It should then be disinfected using the normal procedure (this is because sodium hypochlorite is not effective against spores and cysts of certain organisms).
7. The item may then be safely re-used.

10
Aftercare

Introduction

The purpose of aftercare is to ensure the continued well-being of the patient and in this the practitioner has both reactive and proactive roles. The reactive element involves gathering information, both by conversation with the patient and by clinical observation of the lenses and eyes, and then initiating appropriate management strategies. The proactive element is the encouragement of compliance with lens care that would otherwise deteriorate over time. This second goal is often pursued rather less assiduously than the first, yet it may have a profound influence on the outcome of contact lens wear. To put it another way, prevention is better than cure.

Initially, aftercare appointments could be regarded as part of the fitting process, where minor adjustments are made to the lenses or care system. Once this sequence is complete, the emphasis shifts to the longer-term consequences of lens wear and to keeping the patient both compliant and aware of any developments in lens design or care systems which may be of benefit to them.

Symptoms and history

The first question that should be addressed to any patient presenting for aftercare is: "Are you having any problems, or is this just a routine check?"

If problems are being experienced they are likely to concern discomfort, poor vision or poor cosmetic appearance. For any of these detail is important, and this should always include:

1. Which eye?
2. When did it first start?
3. When does it happen?
4. What seems to set it off?
5. What seems to improve it?
6. Is it getting better or worse?

Discomfort may manifest itself in several ways:

1. If it is felt immediately on insertion it may indicate a sharp or damaged lens edge or a reaction to solutions.
2. If it gradually gets worse over the wearing period, look for evidence of drying and deposition.
3. Pain, as opposed to discomfort, may indicate corneal damage or infection.
4. If the pain gets worse on removal, suspect corneal insult or infection.
5. Photophobia may indicate edema or inflammation.

Poor vision may also appear in several guises:

1. If it is constant, the chances are that the lens power is wrong.
2. If it is poor in one eye only, check that the lenses are in the correct eyes. Most wearers have mixed up their lenses at some point.
3. If it is transient or intermittent, drying of the lens surface – possibly secondary to lens deposits or a poor tear film – is indicated.
4. Vision that gets progressively worse throughout the wearing period may be due to edema or deposits.
5. Spectacle blur, where the vision through spectacles is worse following lens wear, may indicate edema or corneal molding. It should not be noticeable with a well-fitting lens of adequate oxygen transmission though it was a common occurrence with low Dk lenses.
6. If the vision deteriorates over a period of time it may be due to "power creep" where extra minus power is added by over-enthusiastic cleaning. This is more likely to occur if the solution used for cleaning has an abrasive element.

The cause of **redness of the eyes** may be indicated by its distribution:

1. If it is generalized, a solution reaction should be suspected.
2. Drying may cause a band of injected vessels traversing the bulbar conjunctiva from inner to outer canthus.

3. Swollen eyelids and ptosis may be caused by irritation from the lens edge.

Once we know of any problems that will need to be managed, some background information is needed, if we don't already posses it.

The **current lens specification** is important since if we don't know what the patient is using, we won't know how to improve on it. Reception staff should be trained to ask the patient to bring their specification with them to the appointment as the Data Protection Act has made it difficult to gather information from previous practitioners on the day. We should also know the age of the current lenses and the frequency of replacement suggested by the prescribing practitioner.

Previous contact lens history is of interest. If the patient has upgraded their lenses regularly as better ones have become available, it suggests that the general standard of care has been relatively high. Conversely, patients who are wearing lens designs of archaeological interest may be doing so through ignorance of anything better. Those patients who have changed their lens type may have done so in response to problems. The soft lens wearer who converts to RGPs may have had significant neovascularization, and careful slit-lamp examination for ghost vessels is indicated. Where there is a history of repeated inflammatory or infective episodes the likelihood is that the patient is more than usually prone to these events.

We should determine the **pattern of wear** in terms of the number of days per week and the hours per day that the lenses are worn, and whether this is imposed by choice or limited by problems.

The care system needs careful investigation, and a number of questions should be asked:

1. Which solutions are used? It is surprising how few patients actually know the correct name of the solution they are using, and it is useful to keep a few samples in the consulting room as an *aide-mémoire* ("it's that one in the blue bottle on the right").

2. Are these the ones that were prescribed by the practitioner? Surveys have shown that about a third of patients are not using the solutions prescribed, and that the situation deteriorates with time. Patients change for a variety of reasons, including cost, availability and simple curiosity. Some adopt a "pick and mix" approach, using a cleaner from one manufacturer and a conditioning solution from another, and these solutions may not be compatible. Furthermore, if the preservatives are different it can be time-consuming to identify the culprit in the event of solution sensitivity.

3. How old is the case? Patients have a habit of using a case well past its time. This can interfere with the action of the solutions and act as a significant source of infection, particularly as few patients clean cases once the novelty of contact lens wear has worn off.

4. How do you use the solutions? It is best to watch the patient remove their lenses and then clean and disinfect as they normally would (assuming they would). This will give a valuable insight into their general approach to hygiene (did they wash their hands?), lens handling and use of solutions. Patients are often rather creative with solutions. Many clean the lenses before insertion rather than before overnight soaking. "Topping-up" of storage solutions rather than replacement is often adopted as an economy measure, sometimes with unfortunate consequences.

5. Do you use a protein remover? Many patients who have been given protein removers forget to replace them once they run out, or only use them when the lenses start to feel a bit sticky. Infrequent use is ineffective, as denatured protein will not be removed effectively.

6. Have you had any problems with solutions in the past? This will tell us what to avoid in future in case we need to change the solutions in the future.

Vision and over-refraction

In most cases, recording the vision with each eye and binocularly can be followed by a simple spherical over-refraction. If the vision is not correctable to the required standard, sphero-cylindrical refraction may be required. A pinhole can be a quick way to determine whether there is any residual refractive error, and the retinoscope may detect uncorrected astigmatism. It should not be forgotten that contact lens patients are not immune to binocular vision anomalies, and a patient who appears to have good visual acuity who is unhappy with their vision may require binocular investigation.

Assessment of the lenses

The lenses should be examined in situ, first with white light and subsequently with cobalt blue light with fluorescein instilled.

White light investigation with diffuse light, then focal light with an angled beam about 2 mm wide is used to determine the state of the lens. Edge damage and surface deterioration should be apparent. The patient should then be invited to look down and the upper lid raised by the practitioner. As the tear film dries, surface deposits will become apparent:

1. Protein tends to take on a dull, grayish appearance when dried.
2. Lipid deposits are shinier, and look "greasy."

Right-handed patients will sometimes present with the **"left lens syndrome."** The right lens is often cleaned first, and the second lens may not be cleaned quite so thoroughly. In time a significantly higher level of deposition will be seen on the lens that is cleaned second.

Fluorescein should be instilled and the fit of the lenses assessed in the way described in Chapter 4. Practitioners should follow the principle 'if it ain't broke, don't fix it' and resist the urge to fiddle with a fit that is not causing any clinical problems in pursuit of some mythical perfect fit. However, if it is broke, do fix it. If we are going to change anything, there should always be some tangible benefit to the patient, who is probably going to be paying for the change.

The patient should then be asked to remove and store their lenses as normal. While they do this their technique and the state of the case can be observed. Slit-lamp investigation of the patient's eyes can then proceed. This follows the same pattern as that described in Chapter 1, observing the adnexa, tear layer and cornea in sequence.

Management of complications

This will be discussed in Chapter 11.

Promoting compliance

Many contact lens patients do not comply with their wearing schedules or care regimes. This is not a problem specific to contact lenses. Whenever human beings have devised substances or strategies of potential benefit to their fellows, other human beings have found ways of rendering them ineffective or downright dangerous. Non-compliance is not a product of the consumer age either. Hippocrates was moved to opine: "Patients are often lying when they say they have regularly taken their medicine." This may seem a bit harsh, until we consider the facts. For short-term medication, such as a course of antibiotics, non-compliance rates of 20–30% are typical, rising to over 50% when the course of treatment is prolonged. The degree of stubbornness that some patients achieve is staggering. In one study, glaucoma patients were told that they would go blind if they did not comply with medication. Nevertheless, half of them did not comply often enough for the treatment to be effective, and compliance did not improve even after sight was lost in one eye.

A study by Claydon and Efron (1994) gives us some interesting statistics. They found that 27% of patients admitted to wearing their lenses for longer than instructed, and research conducted during the development of silicone hydrogels suggests that many wear unsuitable lenses overnight at least occasionally (this includes RGP wearers). It is also recognized that patients will seek to extend the lifespan of their lenses by using daily disposables for a week or more, and monthlies until they fall apart, often with inadequate care systems.

Claydon and Efron also found significant non-compliance with care systems: 62% keep their solutions for too long, and many of these are probably "topping-up" rather than replacing their solutions daily; 36% clean their lenses only intermittently and 8% not at all; 10% never rinse them. The relationship with tap water is fascinating: 3% consider it a suitable medium for lens cleaning, yet 30% have such an aversion to it that they avoid washing their hands before handling their lenses.

The reasons for non-compliance are manifold. In some cases patients may have been misinformed, either by a practitioner or by acquaintances, or they may have misunderstood the instructions. Simple ignorance should not be discounted. A Bausch & Lomb study found that 35% of patients thought saline was for disinfection, and there is a story (possible apocryphal) of a man who presented in the contact lens clinic of a leading hospital with the complaint that not only were his protein tablets ineffective but that he was sick every time he swallowed one. Cost cutting may motivate some non-compliant behavior. The patient who extends the lifespan of the lenses or of the solution may be penny-pinching but may equally be just too lazy to get some fresh products, and socioeconomic status is a poor predictor of non-compliance.

The effect of boredom should not be ignored. Long-term therapy generally has higher non-compliance rates, and the situation deteriorates the longer the treatment continues. Contact lens care systems fall into the long-term category. Patients run out of a product and either carry on without it or use something else perceived to be similar until they can get to the supplier of the proper stuff. If no adverse effects occur immediately, they have little motivation to return to the original system, especially if the new version is cheaper or easier (and what could be cheaper and easier than doing nothing). Some patients are simply curious. If they see a new product on the shelves of the supermarket they simply have to try it, in the same way they might try out a new shampoo, and advertising encourages such behavior. Finally, there may be some element of risk-compensation involved. We live in a protected world, and some patients, particularly males, may incline towards risky behavior either consciously or subconsciously. After all, we smoke, drink, take recreational drugs and drive above the speed limit, sometimes all at once, despite well-publicized consequences.

Non-compliance may threaten sight. Even when the consequences are more trivial they can waste a considerable amount of chair time, especially as patients rarely make a full confession of their crimes immediately. It is therefore essential that practitioners take steps to maximize compliance, though the statistics do not make encouraging reading.

Patients need to be aware that they are susceptible to complications as a result of non-compliance and that such complications are not rare. Furthermore, the complications are sometimes severe and can result in blindness. While the practitioner would not wish to terrify a patient unnecessarily, when one is faced with an individual whose ambitions appear to encompass the joys of microbial keratitis some shock tactics may be in order. There are many pictures of microbial keratitis available these days, and a suitably gory example, kept on a practice computer or printed out, can concentrate the mind splendidly. Pick one with lots of red bits and purulent discharge for maximum effect. A short discussion of corneal grafts should complete the operation. For less severe transgressions the carrot/stick ratio can be modified by emphasizing the potential benefits to visual performance and comfort of compliant behavior.

Compliance may be aided by ensuring that the care system is simple and quick to use, and easily obtained. Novelty may promote at least short-term compliance, so there is a case for discussing new developments in both lenses and solutions at every aftercare appointment. Free samples of new products are readily available to practitioners and we should make use of them.

The one thing that is generally accepted to promote compliance is repetition. By reminding patients of the correct care regime at aftercare visits Radford et al (1993) found compliance rates could be raised from 44% to 90%.

In summary, the strategy for promoting compliance should begin at the initial consultation and continue throughout the time that the patient continues to wear contact lenses:

1. At the **initial visit,** the practitioner must set an example by washing his or her hands thoroughly before touching either the patient or a lens and by discussing the importance of hygiene and compliance.

2. During the **collection appointment**, clear information on the wearing and care of the lenses needs to be given verbally, although it would be optimistic to expect the patient to listen to it all. Many patients are in a rather nervous and excited state when first collecting their lenses and much of the information goes in one ear and out of the other without ever making any impression on the cognitive centers. For this reason, it is important to back up any verbal information with a written version. It is also useful to get the patient to sign a form acknowledging that a full discussion of the care of the lenses took place, as the patient's memory may be incomplete, especially if things subsequently go wrong.

3. The real work begins at the **first aftercare** visit. The patient should be asked to demonstrate their technique for removal, cleaning and storage of the lenses, and any deficiencies should be addressed. Many patients forget to wash their hands before removing the lenses and this omission should be tackled at an early stage.

4. At subsequent **aftercare** appointments the same procedure should be adopted. We need to know what the patient is using, how they use it and how often they use it. The patient should also be made aware of any developments in lens design or solutions that might be of benefit to them. Too many patients gradually become out of date and eventually turn up for an infrequent aftercare visit wearing lenses that transmit little oxygen, that are worn for too long, and with a care system which is either somewhat minimal or ill-matched to their lenses or wearing pattern. Such behavior becomes ingrained, and it can be difficult to convince such a patient that change is a good thing. The occasional patient who keeps his PMMA lenses on the bathroom shelf and licks them before insertion may prove to be particularly challenging, though it may be worth pointing out that the bacterial load would be lighter if he urinated on them instead!

5. Patients should be encouraged to have regular aftercare at intervals of 6 months to 1 year, as longer periods encourage the patient to get into bad habits. Reminders should be sent out, and if they are not acted upon attempts should be made to contact the patient. It may take up time but it will hopefully avoid the day when the patient turns up with a problem that takes weeks or months to resolve. Planned replacement of the contact lenses will tend to encourage regular attendance, as will the occasional upgrade. Continuity of care should also help in establishing trust between patient and practitioner.

6. It is important that the practitioner keeps abreast of new developments, as advertising in the media and on the internet is far more effective now than it used to be. A practitioner who knows less than the patient will rapidly lose all credibility and their advice will be ignored, probably with some justification. Regular CET and CPD is the remedy, and in the contact lens field the pace of change makes them essential.

References

Claydon BE, Efron N (1994) Non-compliance in contact lens wear. *Ophthal. Physiol. Opt.* **14**:356–64.

Radford CF, Woodward EG, Stapleton F (1993) Contact lens hygiene compliance in a university population. *J. Br. Contact Lens Assoc.* **16**:105–11.

Further Reading

Sokol J, Meir MG, Bloom S (1990) A study of patient compliance in a contact lens wearing population. *Contact Lens Assoc. Ophthalmol. J.* **16**: 209–13.

11

Complications and management

Introduction

Most aftercare appointments are fairly routine affairs and as lens materials, lens designs and the care systems used with them have improved some of the complications that were common have all but disappeared. Nevertheless, from time to time intervention is necessary to resolve problems which have arisen, and we can save time and money for both patient and practitioner by adopting a systematic approach. The strategy for effective management of complications involves the following steps:

1. Know your enemy. Correct identification of the root of the problem will save time and inconvenience. There is a tendency among those new to contact lens aftercare to misidentify the problem, often as a result of an over-reaction to a single clinical finding. Symptoms and signs are rarely solitary and a single finding is rarely specific. The trick is to seek corroborative evidence. The more signs and symptoms that point to the same cause, the more likely it is that the diagnosis is accurate. There are "families" of signs and symptoms and discovery of any family member should always prompt a thorough search for the parents and siblings. For rigid contact lenses, the families are determined by the nature of the lenses themselves. They are hard plastic objects with fairly sharp edges that sit on the eye exerting pressure on the tear layer and cornea and restricting the availability of oxygen. They are accompanied by solutions and deposits which may cause toxic or hypersensitivity reactions. With that in mind, the families are as follow, although there is some overlap between them:
   (a) Hypoxia.
   (b) Drying.
   (c) Mechanical insult.
   (d) Toxic and hypersensitivity reactions.
   (e) Sterile inflammation of the cornea.
   (f) Microbial keratitis.
2. Change one thing at a time; see if it resolves the situation before making any more changes. A scattergun approach may

solve the problem at least as fast, but you won't know why. Should the problem recur, you will be none the wiser how to tackle it.

3. Always keep in mind a worst-case scenario for the sign and symptoms you have collected and an idea of the likely timescale involved. If this involves serious risk to the patient, as it will if microbial keratitis is suspected, make sure that you see the patient again before events can take their course. Bacterial ulcers become serious over hours rather than days, so seeing the patient in a week or so is not sufficient.

4. Unless the worst-case considerations are overriding, allow enough time for the changes to take effect. For example, if the oxygen transmission is improved to eliminate microcysts it makes little sense to see the patient in a fortnight when the microcysts are certain to be more numerous. If the patient is seen in 3 months, you will be able to tell if your management has worked.

5. Try not to just "wait and see." If a finding isn't serious enough to do anything about, it probably won't be in a fortnight either. If it is too serious to ignore, it probably won't improve on its own, although there are always exceptions to every rule. Patients can usually tell if the practitioner is indecisive, and a proactive approach with objectives that are clear to both parties is generally more reassuring. Recording these objectives on the clinical record is essential and if instructions are lengthy then it is worth considering writing them down for the patient.

Hypoxia

All contact lenses restrict the oxygen supply to some extent although, as lenses have developed over the years, the restriction has become much less, and the clinical signs rather more subtle, than in the old days of PMMA lenses, when every patient had central edema visible with the naked eye if the limbus was illuminated. The "family" of signs and symptoms associated with hypoxia include the following.

Symptoms tend to be non-specific if mild, and patients will often complain of dryness when the actual cause is hypoxia. In more severe cases the cornea may become edematous leading to a loss of contrast and light scattering which may cause photophobia towards the end of the wearing period. Central corneal edema may cause steepening. Corneal steepening will cause a myopic shift in the spectacle prescription, though this will be masked during rigid lens wear by the tear lens, which will also increase in minus power. However, if spectacles are worn after the lenses are removed the patient may notice that their distance vision has deteriorated. **Spectacle blur**, while common with PMMA and low-Dk materials, should not be happening with a modern RGP lens. **Corneal steepening** can also be detected by keratometry or photokeratometry, and if the edema is chronic, irregular astigmatism may also be present.

On the slit-lamp, the first sign may be **hyperemia** around the limbus. Corneal signs will depend on the severity of the condition. In extreme cases, edema may be seen as a dense grayish clouding of the central corneal area, best observed using the sclerotic scatter technique described in Chapter 1. With low Dk lenses this may be apparent even with the naked eye. If a patient has this level of edema over a period of time, the central cornea will steepen and become irregular, and the corneal sensitivity will fall. Spectacle blur will be marked, and it may be weeks before the spectacle refraction stabilizes. This "corneal exhaustion syndrome" was quite common at one time, and there are still a few patients wearing low Dk materials who present with it.

For the most part, such extremes are not seen with modern lenses and more subtle signs should be sought. These are similar to those seen in soft lens wearers but the distribution tends to be concentrated under the optic zone of the lens rather than over the whole cornea. The degree of edema present at the time of examination may be indicated by the presence of striae and folds:

1. **Striae** are seen as fine, usually vertical gray-white lines in the posterior stroma. They are best observed in direct illumination

using a parallelepiped beam at about 16–20× magnification, against the background of the pupil area. Striae begin to appear when the level of edema reaches about 5%. In RGP wearers they tend to appear in clusters rather than singly, if the level of edema is sufficiently high. They are probably caused by fluid separation of the collagen fibrils in the posterior stroma, which are predominantly vertically arranged.

2. **Folds** can be observed in the endothelial mosaic using specular reflection, appearing as grooves and ridges. If severe, they may appear as dark branching lines in direct illumination. They are caused by buckling of the posterior stroma with high levels of edema. They appear when the level of edema is about 15% and the cornea is likely to be somewhat hazy when in this state.

Acute hypoxia is probably less significant than **chronic hypoxia**, and the latter may be detected by the following clinical signs:

1. **Epithelial microcysts** and **vacuoles** appear as small gray dots in the epithelium in direct illumination. Initially they may be difficult to tell from dust particles in the tear film, but if the patient blinks they are the ones that do not move. The best way to identify them is to use an angled parallelepiped beam at high (40×) magnification. The area of cornea to observe is that where the indirectly illuminated and retro-illuminated areas meet, that is in **marginal retro-illumination** (Figure 11.1).

2. Microcysts, because they have a higher refractive index than the surrounding tissue, show reversed illumination under these conditions and may appear like tiny pin-pricks. **Vacuoles** are generally slightly bigger and do not show reversed illumination, so they appear as small pimples or bubbles. They represent fluid collected in the intracellular spaces are therefore indicative of edema, which may be caused by hypoxia or hypertonic ocular exposure. It is possible for these intercellular spaces to be exploited by *Acanthamoeba* to gain access to the cornea so the presence of significant numbers should not be tolerated. Some patients may have a few of these independent of contact lens wear. **Microcysts** are probably apoptotic (i.e. dead) cells that are either ingested by

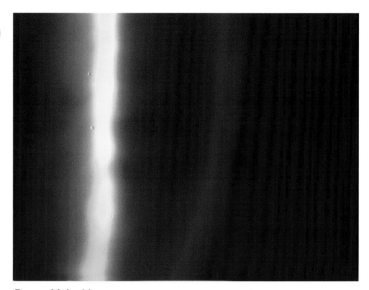

Figure 11.1 Microcysts

phagocytes or encapsulated by material from the basement membrane and eventually expelled after traveling through the corneal layers. They are probably created by a combination of hypoxia, which produces lactic acid, and hypercapnia (increase in carbon dioxide levels), which creates carbonic acid. They may also be induced by mechanical trauma in some cases. They can be eliminated by improving the level of oxygen available, but the recovery process is unusual. Initially, the number of microcysts will increase as the corneal metabolism speeds up and cellular debris is removed more efficiently. There is then a gradual decrease in the number until they are finally eliminated. This can take 3–5 months. The point at which microcysts become significant is subjective, but generally if staining is also present intervention is required.

3. Changes to the endothelium may also occur in response to the acidosis caused by hypoxia and hypercapnia. An acute response is observed in all contact lens wearers within a few

minutes of lens insertion. When the endothelium is observed by the specular reflection a number of dark areas can be observed within the endothelial mosaic. These are **blebs,** and represent swollen cells that disrupt the smooth mirror-like surface of the endothelium/aqueous interface. After 20–30 minutes the number of blebs peaks and thereafter falls over the next hour, though some blebs will be visible throughout the wearing period. The chronic response to acidosis is polymegathism, where the cells of the endothelial mosaic appear to vary markedly in size. **Polymegathism** occurs naturally with age, so the endothelium should be judged against expectations for a given age group. It is not easy to assess the endothelium accurately with a slit-lamp. The highest magnification available is usually 40× or less, and even at 40× with a good slit-lamp the best that can be seen is a textured area, and only the more advanced degrees of polymegathism may be detected with any reliability. This is most likely to be seen with low Dk lenses, especially PMMA, and patients with corneal exhaustion are likely candidates. Polymegathism is a response to significant metabolic stress and remedial action should be taken if it is detected. Recovery is at best very slow, and may not occur at all.

4. Neovascularization is rare as a response to hypoxia in RGP wearers, but not unknown. It is more likely if the lens is decentered or binding in such a way as to cover the area adjacent to the limbus and if low Dk materials are used.

Significant chronic hypoxia is known to increase the risk of microbial keratitis, and it is now easy to address. The **management of hypoxia**, unsurprisingly, consists of arranging for greater oxygen availability. This may be achieved by the following strategies:

1. Wearing the lenses less. This may be effective in the short term, but rarely in the longer term. The wearing pattern that a patient adopts is largely dictated by convenience to that individual and the patient will probably return to their previous wearing pattern sooner rather than later.

2. Improving the flow of tears under the lens may improve oxygen levels to a limited extent. A smaller total diameter, greater edge lift and smoother transitions may bring some improvement.

3. By far the most effective strategy is to use a more permeable material. There are materials available now that have sufficient permeability to eliminate signs of hypoxia in any normal cornea. It should be borne in mind, if microcysts are being used as an indicator, that refitting with a high Dk material will initially *increase* the number, so an aftercare interval of about 3 months is useful unless contraindicated by other clinical concerns.

Drying

Many patients complain of symptoms of dryness, but not all of them are actually due to drying. Considerable research has been undertaken in recent years with a view to improving the wetting performance of contact lenses but the improvement in patient satisfaction, while considerable, has been less than perhaps anticipated. What patients are actually complaining of is persistent, progressive mild irritation and lens awareness, and this could be due to hypoxia or mild inflammation rather than drying per se.

Drying can cause lens awareness or discomfort, and this usually worsens progressively throughout the wearing time. The vision is often variable due to the accumulation of deposits on the lens, and again this gets worse towards the end of the wearing period. The other frequent patient complaint is of red eyes, and characteristically this is associated with hyperemia of the bulbar conjunctiva in the area exposed between the lid margins.

Clinical signs to look for include the following.

Anomalies of the lid margin. These are best viewed by diffuse illumination under fairly low magnification and they may give a clue to the underlying cause of the problem. **Blepharitis**, which can be associated with changes in both conjunctiva and

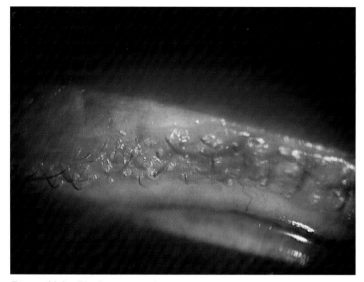

Figure 11.2 Blepharitis

cornea, may cause an unstable tear film that could affect contact lens wear (Figure 11.2).

Chronic blepharitis may be encountered as the anterior form, either staphylococcal or seborrheic. There is also a posterior type, also known as meibomian gland dysfunction. The **staphylococcal** form tends to be seen in patients with atopic eczema and is more common in females and young patients. The lid margins are hyperemic and show telangiectases (dilated, tortuous blood vessels). There is also scaling. The scales are brittle and form collarettes around the bases of the lashes. Where they have been removed, small bleeding ulcers may be seen. This condition is caused by chronic staphylococcal infection of the bases of the lashes, so any patient with it has an increased bacterial load. It should be eliminated before contact lens wear is allowed. Complications that may be observed include whitening or complete loss of the lashes and trichiasis. The lid margins may become scarred and notched. If the infection spreads to the glands of Zeis and Moll a stye may be the result. If the meibomian glands become involved there may be an internal hordeolum. Acute bacterial conjunctivitis may appear, and recur. Apart from these direct bacterial effects, the exotoxins released by the bacteria may cause hypersensitivity reactions. A mild papillary conjunctivitis, marginal corneal infiltrates or, rarely, phlyctenulosis and pannus may occur. About half of all sufferers also have an unstable tear film. Management consists of lid scrubs and referral to a general medical practitioner for antibiotics and possibly anti-inflammatory agents.

The **seborrheic** version tends to be associated with seborrhoeic dermatitis which can affect the scalp, face and chest. There is an oily type in which the scaling is greasy, and also a dry type (dandruff). The symptoms are similar to, though milder than, the staphylococcal form. The hyperemia and telangiectasia of the lid margins are also more moderate, and the scales are greasy and yellowish and do not leave an ulcer when removed. The lids may be greasy and stuck together. There may be a moderate papillary conjunctivitis and punctate keratitis, which tends to favor the middle third of the cornea, whereas the staphylococcal form often affects the lower third of the cornea. Management usually involves lid scrubs, using sodium bicarbonate as a de-greasing agent.

Posterior blepharitis (meibomian gland dysfunction, MGD) may be divided into meibomian seborrhea and meibomitis. Meibomian seborrhea causes hypersecretion from dilated meibomian glands. The lid margins may show small oil globules or waxy collections. The tear film may be oily and foamy and in severe cases there may be a frothy discharge at the inner canthus (meibomian foam). The patient complains of burning eyes on first waking but there may be few signs of inflammation, so this is easy to miss. If the lid margins are gently squeezed copious discharge may be elicited. It should be remembered that the lid margins are sensitive, and the expression of meibomian contents usually hurts, especially when attempted by the inexperienced. It is therefore not a procedure to be recommended on an asymptomatic patient.

Primary meibomitis involves inflammation centered around the orifices of the meibomian glands, which may pout and be capped by domes of oily material (meibomana). Expressed meibomian contents are thickened and may contain more solid particles, in some cases resembling toothpaste and requiring firm pressure to express. If the contents become trapped, meibomian cysts may form. Papillary conjunctivitis and punctate epitheliopathy may be secondary effects. About a third of these patients have tear film instability. Meiobomitis may also occur with secondary seborrheic blepharitis, associated with seborrheic dermatitis, the meibomian involvement usually being relatively mild and patchy. Management involves lid scrubs and referral to the patient's general medical practitioner for oral antibiotics, typically tetracycline. Treatment may take 3 months or more.

The contact lenses are likely to have heavy **deposits** of protein, lipid or both. The exact nature of the deposits will depend on individual tear chemistry, the lens material and the solution being used. If the upper lid is held by the practitioner and the patient instructed to look down, the surface of the lens will dry. Protein deposits tend to have a dull, grayish appearance whereas lipid deposits are shinier. The pre-lens tear film is likely to be unstable.

Following lens removal, other signs may be apparent:

1. The tear break-up time (TBUT) may be low, often below 10 seconds, and the tear layer will appear foamy or "bitty."
2. The bulbar conjunctiva will be hyperemic, usually in a band from inner to outer canthus. Frequently, there will be marked conjunctival fluorescein staining in the same area. In severe cases a wing-shaped vascular lesion may encroach upon the cornea from the conjunctiva. This is **pseudopterygium** rather than true pterygium, which is a degenerative condition, although it may look similar.
3. There may be corneal staining. High-riding, lid-attached lenses often cause inferior corneal stain outside the area covered by the lens edge. Lower-riding lenses tend to cause **3 and 9 o'clock stain** (Figure 11.3). A small amount of this is common, but if severe, the underlying stromal layers may desiccate and become compacted. This leads to saucer-shaped depressions in the cornea (**dellen**). Initially at least the

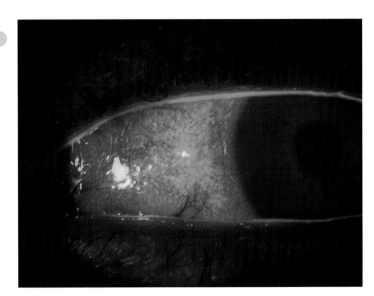

Figure 11.3 Severe 3 and 9 o'clock staining with extended interpalpebral desiccation (courtesy of D. Ruston)

epithelium may be intact, but over time scarring and vascularization may occur.

Management of dryness can involve a number of strategies:

1. Elimination of causative factors, especially the various forms of blepharitis, should be pursued. Lid scrubs and hot compresses will be useful for MGD and seborrheic anterior blepharitis, while staphylococcal blepharitis will need antimicrobial treatment which may require routine referral to a general medical practitioner. However, if the dryness of the eyes is caused by systemic medication or a medical condition, elimination of the cause may be outside the control of the contact lens practitioner.

2. Careful selection of care systems may help to reduce or remove deposits. Lipid deposits are often seen with solutions containing chlorhexidene. Protein deposition may require the

use of an enzyme cleaner. Compliance with cleaning regimes
should also be encouraged.

3. Old lenses tend to deposit more, so planned replacement may
help considerably, particularly with modern materials which
tend to scratch more easily.

4. The use of surface-treated lenses or hybrid materials may
improve comfort considerably as well as reducing deposition.

5. If all else fails, rewetting or "comfort" drops may relieve
symptoms. However, they are rarely a long-term solution as
patients often eventually either stop using them or use them
so infrequently that they make little difference. In the past, a
few patients went to the other extreme, instilling copious
amounts of preserved comfort drops and eventually becoming
allergic to them.

Mechanical insult

RGP lenses are fairly rigid and have relatively sharp edges, so
mishandling on insertion and removal may cause corneal insult.
Once the lens is on the cornea it may cause mechanical stress on
a number of tissues:

1. Compression of the central cornea, sometimes associated with
lens flexure, appears as a polygonal mosaic staining pattern.
This is known as a Fischer–Schweitzer pattern and is more
common after overnight wear. It usually disappears a few hours
after waking.

2. Steep lenses may trap small bubbles under the optic zone.
These can cause small circular depressions in the cornea which
may retain fluorescein even though the epithelial surface is
intact. With the major slit-lamp it looks like rather coarse and
neatly circular punctate staining. This **dimple veiling** is usually
asymptomatic, though if severe some visual degradation may be
noticed. A flatter fit, increased edge lift or smoother transitions
will generally eliminate it. Dimple veil can also be associated with
mucin balls. These are created by sheer forces acting on
the mucin component of the tears and with the lens in place

appear as small gray bodies between the back surface of the lens and the cornea. Though more often associated with soft lenses, mucin balls are fairly common with some RGP materials. They rarely cause problems but there are reports of a correlation between mucin balls and an increased frequency of inflammatory events.

3. RGP lenses may **bind** onto the cornea. This is a common occurrence in overnight wear, though it may also be observed occasionally in conventional wear. The lens is usually decentered laterally or downwards. A circular indentation of the cornea may be caused by the lens edge. Superficial punctate keratitis may be seen in the circular pattern adjacent to the compression ring, or centrally within it. The cause may be multifactorial. Loss of the aqueous component of the tear film will produce a viscous, mucin-rich tear film which effectively glues the lens to the eye. Surface deposits, particularly protein hazing of silicone acrylate materials, have also been implicated. Suction effects associated with lens flexure that some high transmission lenses are prone to may also result in a bound lens. Finally, in overnight wear, the peak time for adherence appears to correlate with the peak of the diurnal variation in intraocular pressure. It is possible that this causes lateral stresses making binding more likely. A bound lens may be uncomfortable and the vision may be poor if decentered, but many patients have few symptoms. Lens adhesion is common in RGP extended wear, and patients should be instructed to check for it every morning. The use of rewetting drops and digital manipulation of the lens will help the occasional adhered lens, but persistent binding should be tackled if the patient is to continue extended wear, as it may lead to corneal distortion, vascularization and ulceration. Management of binding may involve changes to the lens or the care system. A smaller lens with a wide, flat periphery will improve tear exchange and is less likely to approach the corneal surface. Conversely, a steeper BOZR may reduce the contact area over which mucus adhesion can occur, although it may lead to increased lens flexure. A change in care system may help. It has been reported that changing patients from

Boston Advance conditioning solution to the original Boston solution reduced the incidence of binding. For those patients prone to surface deposits, an abrasive cleaner and/or enzyme cleaner may prove effective, provided that they use it regularly. However, planned replacement of the lenses at 3–6 month intervals is likely to be more effective as it does not rely as much on patient compliance.

4. Edge irritation may be caused by a sharp edge profile or by a damaged edge, often caused when the lens is dropped. The edge is best inspected with a slit-lamp, and some idea of its profile may be obtained by looking at the reflex created by the light source. Too narrow a reflex indicates a sharp edge, and this may cause problems particularly if the apex is towards the front of the edge profile. Chronic irritation may produce **ptosis**, which will generally resolve on cessation of lens wear.

5. Mechanical irritation may also induce **papillary conjunctivitis**, usually of the upper lid. The earliest sign is hyperemia of the upper palpebral conjunctiva relative to conjunctiva of the lower lid, though this may be asymptomatic. Later papillae will appear and may coalesce to form giant papillae with diameters over 1 mm. The papillae themselves are hyperplastic vascular tissue and have a central vascular core. Should the papillae become inflamed, the lens may adhere to them and decenter, creeping up under the lid. With RGP lenses, the response often appears first near the lid margins and progresses towards the fornices. It may also be caused by an immune response to deposits on the lens. Management will depend on the perceived cause. Mechanical papillary conjunctivitis may be tackled by improving the edge profile, reducing edge stand-off by changing the total diameter or reducing edge lift in one or more meridians. That due to deposits may be improved by more effective cleaning and frequent lens replacement.

Toxic and hypersensitivity reactions

Intolerance to solutions is considerably less common than was once the case, due to improvements in their formulation, particularly to the preservative elements. However, hypersensitivity reactions are still encountered from time to time. Some become apparent within a day or two of first use of the solution, but there are occasions when the symptoms gradually build up over a period of time before they become severe enough for the patient to consult their practitioner. Early clinical signs may be apparent in an asymptomatic patient. The symptoms associated with solution intolerance are typically noticed immediately after the lenses are inserted and may resolve if the lenses are kept in and the solutions diluted by the tear film. Lens awareness, itching, burning and sensations of dryness are all common. In severe cases photophobia may be reported.

In patients with mild or no symptoms, the clinical signs may include the following:

1. Hyperemia of the palpebral and bulbar conjunctiva. The latter may be in a diffuse pattern or more marked around the limbus.
2. Superficial punctate keratitis (SPK). This may favor the lower cornea, but is typically diffused over the corneal surface.
3. Occasionally, infiltrates may be observed. These are usually intraepithelial or subepithelial. They may be discrete or diffuse, and tend to favor the area just inside the limbus.

More severe reactions will have symptoms, sometimes quite marked, and the following signs may be present:

1. The lids may be swollen.
2. The tear film may be unstable and mucus strands may be visible. Reflex lacrimation is common.
3. Conjunctival hyperemia.
4. Diffuse SPK.
5. In hypersensitivity reactions, infiltrates may be observed, though there is usually a delay of about 24 hours between the initial signs and symptoms and the appearance of infiltrates.

The management of solution reactions will depend on their severity. If the symptoms and signs are severe, it is wise to suspend contact lens wear until the eye returns to normal, especially as the signs of microbial infection may be rather similar. If there is any question of infection, the patient should be seen the next day. Once the initial reaction has subsided, or if the clinical signs are mild to begin with, management involves identifying likely triggering agents and avoiding them. The prime suspect in these cases is usually the preservative in the conditioning solution. However, a surprising number of patients clean their lenses before insertion and may not rinse them thoroughly, so the cleaning solution may also be a factor to consider. Buffering agents and residues from enzymatic systems may also be suspected on occasion. Careful questioning of the patient is necessary to establish precisely what solutions are in use, and how they are used. It may not even be the solutions used for the lenses, as self-prescribed or medical practitioner-prescribed eye-drops can cause the same reactions. Where more than one potential suspect is present eliminate them one at a time, in descending order of probability, until the signs and symptoms are eliminated. Strictly speaking, a causal relationship can only be proven by reintroducing the suspected agent and observing the return of clinical signs. However, this may be a test too far for most contact lens wearers and so this step is usually omitted.

Sterile inflammation of the cornea

Inflammation of the cornea is not specific to one causative agent. The same response will occur whatever the initial trigger. The trigger can be trauma, toxicity or immune response and the common factor is that corneal cells, usually in the epithelium, become distressed and release chemical agents which initiate the inflammatory response. Rigid contact lens wear tends to potentiate all of the likely triggers:

1. **Trauma** is more likely as the cornea may be hypoxic, which makes the epithelium more fragile and slow to repair. RGP

lenses are hard and sharp objects which have potential to cause physical trauma if mishandled.

2. Contact lens solutions, deposits and bacterial toxins are all capable of inducing a **toxic response**. In extended wear, the products of dead epithelial cells may also be a source, though this is less of a problem in extended wear with RGPs than with soft lenses.

3. Solutions, deposits and bacterial toxins may also cause immune responses and the cornea may also react to chemicals released by adjacent inflamed tissues such as the palpebral conjunctiva. Infiltrates are sometimes noted as an **"innocent bystander" effect** of contact lens-related papillary conjunctivitis.

Inflammation consists of four classic elements: rubor, calor, tumor and dolor. Vascular dilation causes (i) rubor (redness or hyperemia) and (ii) calor (increase in temperature), while increased vascular permeability results in (iii) tumor (swelling, edema) and (iv) dolor (discomfort and pain).

In the anterior eye these signs are often fairly subtle unless the response is severe, and a severe response always suggests the possibility of infection. In the cornea, the most useful sign of inflammation is the presence of infiltrates, which are collections of white blood cells. These may form discrete patches or diffuse areas in the epithelium and anterior stroma. Generally speaking, the more serious the cause, the deeper they are and the more likely they are to be central, but this is only a rough guide.

Clinically, corneal infiltrates can be divided into the following categories, in ascending order of seriousness:

1. Asymptomatic infiltrates (AI).
2. Asymptomatic infiltrative keratitis (AIK).
3. Infiltrative keratitis (IK).
4. Contact lens associated red eye (CLARE).
5. Contact lens peripheral ulcer (CLPU).
6. Microbial keratitis (MK, see page 180 under 'Infection').

Asymptomatic infiltrates are sometimes seen in non-contact lens wearers (about 5%), and are probably unrelated to contact lens wear as they have a similar incidence in contact lens wearers. They may be induced by environmental factors such as air

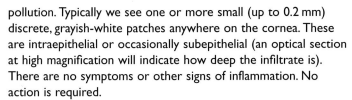

pollution. Typically we see one or more small (up to 0.2 mm) discrete, grayish-white patches anywhere on the cornea. These are intraepithelial or occasionally subepithelial (an optical section at high magnification will indicate how deep the infiltrate is). There are no symptoms or other signs of inflammation. No action is required.

In **asymptomatic infiltrative keratitis** there is a diffuse infiltrate in the peripheral parts of the cornea, sometimes with some discrete infiltrates as well. It doesn't appear to cause any problems in itself, but it may be a mild form of CLARE, with similar causes, so the patient's lens care routine should be under scrutiny.

Infiltrative keratitis can present as a diffuse or focal infiltrate but here it is accompanied by symptoms of discomfort or pain and by bulbar conjunctival hyperemia, especially around the limbal area. The focal form is probably a response to local epithelial trauma caused by a foreign body trapped under an immobile lens. The diffuse form may be a mild form of CLARE response, with similar etiology.

Contact lens red eye (CLARE) itself is a complication of extended wear, and typically the onset is in the early hours of the morning, after a period when the eyes have been closed. It is less common with RGP lenses than soft, but it has been reported with bound, immobile lenses. There is an association with gram-negative bacteria as about a third of CLARE cases have contaminated lenses. The symptoms vary from mild discomfort to pain and there is marked bulbar hyperemia, especially around the limbus. Faint diffuse infiltrates are seen arising from the limbal arcades, though there may be focal infiltrates present as well.

Contact lens peripheral ulcer (CLPU) presents as a round or oval grayish-white infiltrate with an overlying full-thickness epithelial defect. It is generally located near the periphery of the cornea, though there is a band of clear cornea between the infiltrate and the limbus. These ulcers may be asymptomatic or painful. Hyperemia may be generalized or limited to an area adjacent to the lesion. They are culture negative, although a correlation has been found with high levels of gram-positive bacteria. If lens wear is suspended signs and symptoms will resolve in 48 hours except for the infiltrate which can persist up to 3 months, although it usually resolves within 1 month. It is likely that the infiltrate represents a response to localized trauma or toxicity and that the epithelial loss is a result of leukocyte action. However, given the epithelial defect and the bacterial correlation, caution is advisable, and the patient should be seen the next morning if they are not referred.

The management of sterile inflammation depends both on its severity and on the chances that it might be an infection. The asymptomatic and white-eyed forms generally need no intervention, although CLARE's smaller sisters might be regarded as a warning shot from the bacteria and lens hygiene might be worth some scrutiny. The symptomatic forms will require suspension of lens wear. This should ideally be until infiltrates have resolved, unless we are sure that the cause is unthreatening. The time required will vary with the location and depth of the infiltrate. Intraepithelial infiltrates resolve within 2–3 weeks, but subepithelial and anterior stromal ones take longer, up to 3 months in some cases. Anything that persists longer than that in the absence of active inflammation is probably a scar, and these tend to have a "bulls-eye" appearance, with a fainter center.

Infection

The eye may be infected by viruses, fungi, bacteria and amebae, but it is only the last two that can be considered contact lens complications. Wearers may present with viral or fungal infection but it is unlikely that their contact lenses played a significant part in the etiology. However, in bacterial and amoebic infection contact lens wear is a significant risk factor and the majority of patients presenting at eye emergency departments for these conditions are contact lens wearers. The precise incidence of microbial keratitis is difficult to pin down since cultures are unreliable and many patients are treated as infectious cases on appearance rather than waiting for the unpleasant later stages to confirm the diagnosis. An incidence of between 0.012% and 0.07% has been suggested for RGP lenses worn on a daily basis, although figures for extended wear are rather higher.

Rigid contact lenses modify the flushing action of the tears and may change the mucin layer of the tear film. They restrict the oxygen supply to a greater or lesser extent. A hypoxic epithelium is less resistant to abrasion and slower to repair. Microorganisms adhere more easily to the cornea when oxygen levels are low. Finally, both the contact lenses and the storage case may be carrying far more microorganisms than would normally be present in the eye. The most common infections by far are bacterial. In non-contact lens wearers, gram-positive bacteria such as *Staphylococcus* are the most common ocular infectors, but contact lens wear appears to favor gram-negative bacteria, particularly *Pseudomonas aeruginosa*. The fact that the active form of *Acanthamoeba* feeds on gram-negative bacteria may suggest why it is almost exclusively a problem encountered in contact lens wearers.

The **PEDAL** (pain, epithelial defect, discharge, anterior chamber activity, location) mnemonic is widely used when attempting to differentiate between sterile and microbial (especially bacterial) keratitis. However, in contact lens wearers it has some limitations:

1. **Pain** may vary considerably between individuals but in general, the worse it is the more likely it is that we are dealing with an infection. However, there are some patients whose corneal sensitivity is reduced (patients with corneal fatigue and those who have had corneal surgery) and it is not uncommon to see long-term PMMA wearers with scars that suggest bacterial ulcers who have no recollection of what should have been a rather painful episode.
2. An **epithelial defect** overlying an infiltrate is always worrying, although it may be caused by the actions of white blood cells rather than by an infecting microbe. However, many "sterile" inflammations are associated with bacterial toxins and the combination of high levels of bacteria and a breached epithelium is one which leaves considerable scope for secondary infection.

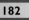
3. **Discharge** is rather variable. *Staphylococcus* may produce little or no discernible discharge. *Streptococcus* and the gram-negative bacteria tend to be fairly gooey, and gonorrhea highly productive.
4. **Anterior chamber activity** should always be present during active ulceration but it varies from a trace to dense flare and cells. Sterile lesions (e.g. CLARE) may also be associated with a moderate anterior chamber reaction.
5. **Location** is also somewhat unreliable in contact lens wearers. In non-wearers, ulcers tend to favor the central areas of the cornea, remote from the limbal vasculature. However, this is not the case in contact lens wearers, as their corneas are more likely to have physical damage peripherally and the virulent organisms involved are able to overcome the ocular defenses. For a contact lens wearer, any suspicious staining lesion in the central area is quite possibly an ulcer, but more peripheral ones could also be ulcers.

When attempting to diagnose a **bacterial infection** it is useful to consider **risk factors**. Contact lens related factors include:

1. Non-compliance with care regimes.
2. Poor hygiene.
3. Lens binding.
4. Extended wear.
5. Old lenses (> 6 months).
6. Dirty lenses.
7. Dirty case.

In addition there are some **health-related factors** that will increase the chances of infection:

1. Diabetes.
2. Travel to a warm climate.
3. Staphylococcal toxins (blepharitis and marginal infiltrates).
4. Dry eyes.
5. Immunocompromised patients (e.g. AIDS patients or those on immune suppressant drugs).

6. Post-surgical corneas.
7. Use of topical steroids.
8. Corneal trauma.

In general it is thought that bacteria are unable to infect a cornea with an intact epithelium although some strains of *Pseudomonas* are capable of this in laboratory conditions at least.

The signs and symptoms of bacterial infection are a combination of effects attributable to the organism and its associated toxins and those produced by the opposing defense mechanisms, which may in some cases be rather worse.

Symptoms may vary according to individual tolerance but include (in approximate ascending order of seriousness):

1. Irritation or lens awareness.
2. Burning sensation, often associated with bacterial toxins.
3. Lacrimation.
4. Photophobia secondary to edema.
5. Reduced VA secondary to edema and infiltration.
6. Foreign body sensation, especially if it increases upon lens removal.
7. Dull aching pain due to inflammation and uveal involvement.

Clinical signs will also vary according to the bacterial strain involved. They include the following:

1. The lids may be swollen and a pseudoptosis may be present.
2. The palpebral conjunctiva will have a red, "meaty" appearance and papillae will be present.
3. Mucopurulent discharge will be present in the tears, especially with streptococcal and gram-negative bacterial infection.
4. The bulbar conjunctiva will be purplish-red and often swollen. Hemorrhages are sometimes seen with streptococcal and gram-negative infections.
5. Corneal ulceration destroys the epithelium and underlying stroma, producing a depressed lesion. This may be clearly defined (typical of streptococci) or indistinct around the edges, and the margins may show an overhang of tissue.

Fluorescein stain will pool in the depression and fluoresce brightly but will then spread into the stroma amorphously within minutes.

6. A lesion over 2 mm in diameter should be regarded as microbial, but they all have to start somewhere and smaller lesions should not be discounted on dimensions alone.

7. The corneal stroma will become edematous, often involving more than 50% of the area and depth.

8. Infiltration will be deep, sometimes full thickness, and will be seen as a hazy or opaque area. Occasionally a deep ring infiltrate is seen with *Pseudomonas*.

9. Stromal abscess, stromal melting and perforation can occur with virulent forms, sometimes within a day or two.

10. Anterior chamber activity may range from very mild to severe cells and flare, sometimes forming an hypopyon in the anterior chamber. The intraocular pressure may increase secondary to anterior chamber involvement, although it might be a bit of a challenge to measure it.

11. The pupil is often miotic.

12. Neovascularization may occur if treatment is delayed.

13. Scarring of the corneal stroma is more or less inevitable.

The time it takes for things to get serious will vary with the organism involved, but the more virulent forms of *Pseudomonas* can cause severe scarring or perforation within a day or two. With this in mind, if corneal infection is suspected it is wise to see the patient the next day, preferably in the morning, if you haven't already referred them to the emergency department of the local eye hospital. If there is more than a suspicion, this should be treated as an ocular emergency and referred without delay.

Acanthamoeba is a common protozoan which occasionally produces severe corneal problems, almost invariably in contact lens wearers. It exists in both an active trophozoite form and as an inert, highly resistant cyst. Though most often associated with soft lenses, *Acanthamoeba* keratitis (AK) has been found in RGP wearers. It is known that exposure to stagnant water sources will increase risk, and these include swimming pools, hot tubs and the

domestic hot water supply. There is often, but not always, a
history of corneal trauma.

The symptoms are not specific to *Acanthamoeba,* but the pain
reported is often far more dramatic than the clinical findings
would suggest. Early clinical signs include:

1. Swollen lids.
2. Perilimbal hyperemia.
3. Staining at this stage is often minimal, but it fails to respond to
   standard anti-infective regimes.

Later signs include:

1. Corneal infiltrates, which tend to mimic those of other
   conditions, leading to misdiagnosis. They may be nummular,
   mimicking adenovirus, or pseudodendritic in form which may
   lead to a diagnosis of herpes simplex or zoster. Other "viral"
   signs such as pseudomembranes and pre-auricular adenopathy
   may be present. Any patient diagnosed with these conditions
   who fails to respond to treatment may have AK.
2. Perilimbal infiltrates are specific to *Acanthamoeba*, and may
   account for the excessive pain associated with this condition.
3. A ring infiltrate or ulcer will eventually form. Stromal melt and
   perforation are possible.
4. Anterior chamber activity may be marked, and hypopyon and
   scleral melt are possible.

The condition advances slowly in comparison to bacterial events,
often with remissions. It is difficult to identify positively and
treatment is often initiated ex juvantia (i.e. when other therapy
has failed). When correct treatment is initiated it may take
months to resolve and the prognosis may be poor.

Where *Acanthamoeba* is suspected (and it should always be
suspected if the pain is disproportionate to the clinical signs, or if
the condition has failed to resolve as expected), prompt referral
is indicated. As a temporary measure, Brolene (propamidine
isetionate) has been found to have a limited action against the
active form.

Index